Bakerita

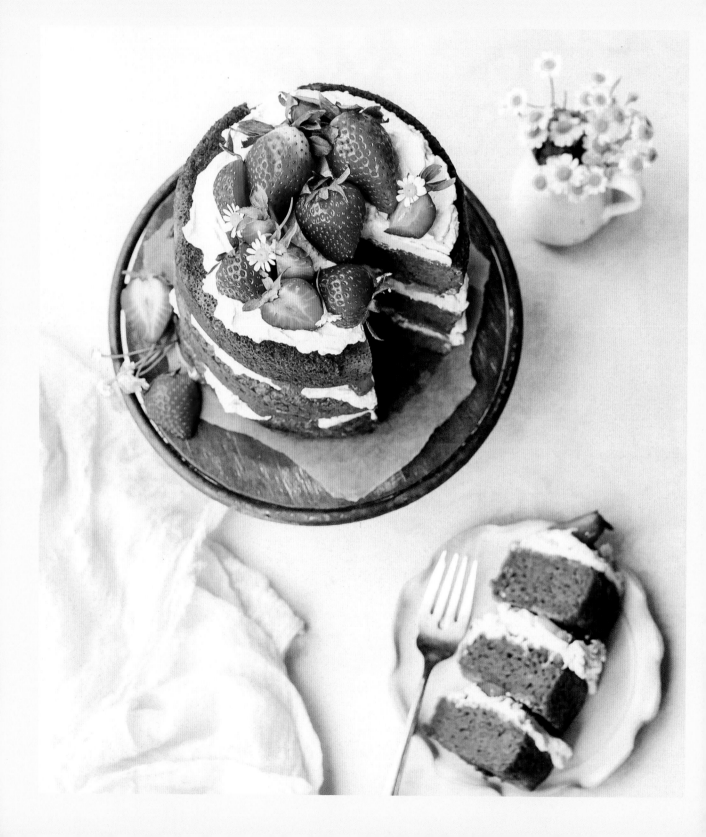

Bakerita

100+ NO-FUSS GLUTEN-FREE, DAIRY-FREE, AND REFINED SUGAR-FREE RECIPES FOR THE MODERN BAKER

RACHEL CONNERS
with Mary Goodbody

HOUGHTON MIFFLIN HARCOURT
BOSTON NEW YORK 2020

For information about permission to reproduce selections from this book, write to trade.permissions@hmhco.com or to Permissions, Houghton Mifflin Harcourt Publishing Company, 3 Park Avenue, 19th Floor, New York, New York 10016.

hmhbooks.com

Library of Congress Cataloging-in-Publication Data

Names: Conners, Rachel, author. | Goodbody, Mary, author.
Title: Bakerita : 100+ no-fuss gluten-free, dairy-free, and refined sugar-free recipes for
    the modern baker / Rachel Conners with Mary Goodbody.
Description: Boston : Houghton Mifflin Harcourt, 2020. | Includes index.
Identifiers: LCCN 2019033897 (print) | LCCN 2019033898 (ebook) |
    ISBN 9780358116677 (pap) | ISBN 9780358116660 (ebook)
Subjects: LCSH: Baking. | Desserts. | Gluten-free diet—Recipes. | LCGFT: Cookbooks.
Classification: LCC TX765 .C63 2020 (print) | LCC TX765 (ebook) | DDC 641.81/5—dc23
LC record available at https://lccn.loc.gov/2019033897
LC ebook record available at https://lccn.loc.gov/2019033898

Book design by Allison Chi

Printed in China

TOP 10 9 8 7 6 5 4 3 2 1

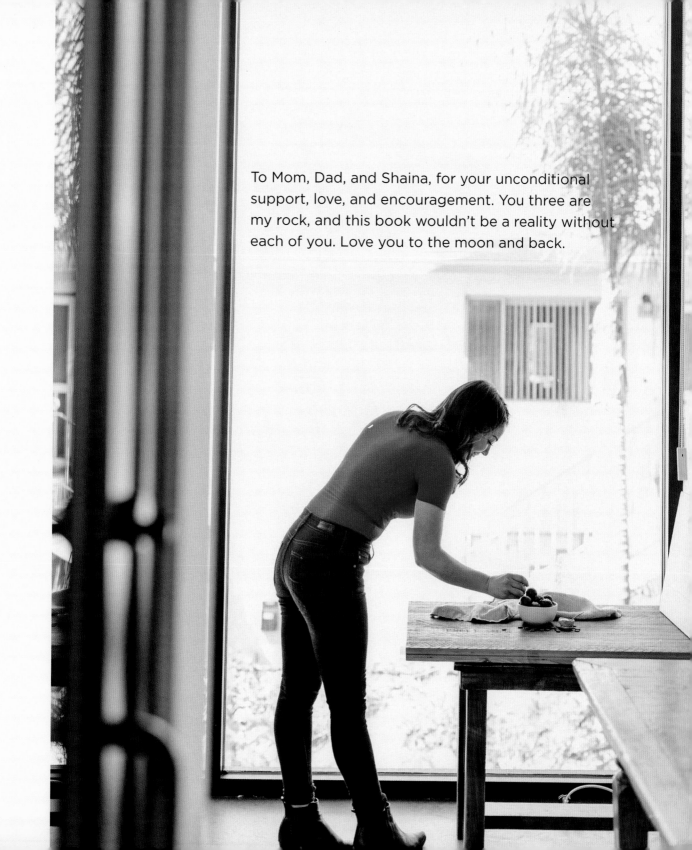

To Mom, Dad, and Shaina, for your unconditional support, love, and encouragement. You three are my rock, and this book wouldn't be a reality without each of you. Love you to the moon and back.

Table of Contents

Acknowledgments

To my *Bakerita* community: I am in awe—your support over the past ten years of *Bakerita*'s existence has allowed me to follow my passion and turn it into a career. This is all for you, and I am so happy you are a part of my life and this journey.

Shaina, thank you for being my constant teacher and guide. *Bakerita* wouldn't exist without you, and I couldn't be more grateful for the inspiration and support you give me in every aspect of my life. You are the best sister, friend, and role model. I'm forever thankful for our relationship.

Mom, thank you for being my original baking teacher and constant cheerleader. You have always been there for me on my hardest days, and I know I can turn to you for anything and everything. You have shown me how to be my best self and given me all I could've dreamt of.

Dad, thank you for always encouraging me to follow this path and instilling in me that whatever it was I chose to do in this world, if I loved it, I would succeed. Thank you for always supporting me with your words and love, and for always allowing me to make your kitchen a mess, even though you hate having a messy kitchen. I am so grateful for you.

Kyle, thank you for being unconditionally supportive, despite coming into my life at such a crazy time. Thank you for tasting nearly everything in this book and giving me honest feedback on all it (and even telling me when certain photos weren't my best . . . and then encouraging me to reshoot them so one could eventually become the cover of the book). I am forever grateful for you as my partner, friend, and guide.

Grammy, Pop Pop, Chini, and Hugo, thank you all for creating a family that loves boundlessly and supports endlessly. I am so grateful for your wisdom, guidance, and love.

Patty, John, Veronica, Tony, Sophia, Maya, and Isabella: You are my favorite travel buddies and my best gluten-eating recipe critics. I can't wait for our next adventure.

Lori, Brian, Sami, Tara, Nir, Zachy, Max, Jordan, Eliana, Steven, Matthew, and Spencer: You all never cease to make me smile and can always lift me up on bad days. Thank you for being my best recipe tasters and for always giving your most honest feedback (especially you little ones).

Paige, my original baking buddy and forever friend: I couldn't be more grateful for your creativity, love, and support. Your texts full of recipe ideas always make me smile, and I'll never forget you holding up bedsheets to serve as my photo backgrounds in the early days. Every cookie dough recipe I ever make is dedicated to you!

Monica of *The Movement Menu*, thank you for being my first food blogger friend in San Diego! I am so grateful for your friendship, guidance, and kinship in this crazy world.

Lindsay of *Weeknight Bite*, thank you for always making me laugh and smile with your recipe feedback videos with Mitch. So grateful to have you as a friend, and for testing all my cookie recipes for me!

Meg of *Nutmeg & Honeybee*, thank you for allowing me to be my full self with you. I am so grateful for the positive impact your friendship has had on my life.

Maddie and Tiffany, I had no idea the day we planned our first photo shoot that those photos would end up throughout my first cookbook. Thank you for capturing me (and Hank!) with your amazing photo skills!

Mary, thank you for your organization, support, recipe-testing skills, and constant feedback as we tested every recipe in this book to make sure it was perfect. You kept me sane!

Leigh Eisenman, I am eternally grateful for your support and guidance during the entire book process. This cookbook wouldn't exist in its current form without you. Thank you for always staying positive when it seemed as if things were going sideways and reminding me that better things are to come. You were right!

Justin Schwartz, my editor at Houghton Mifflin Harcourt, thank you for seeing my vision and helping me turn my dream of a *Bakerita* cookbook into a reality.

Allison Chi, thank you for designing the *Bakerita* cookbook to be as beautiful as I ever could have imagined!

To the entire team at HMH, I am so grateful to all of you for cocreating this book with me. Thank you for all of your work and insights.

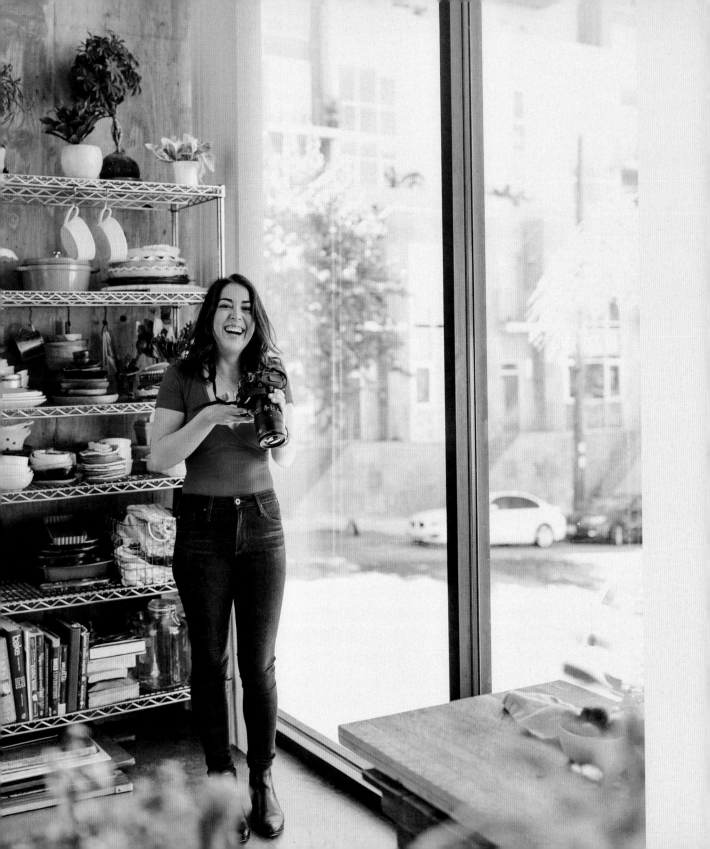

My Story

AS A YOUNG GIRL, my eyes were always fixed on the sweets in whatever room I was in, particularly anything with chocolate or peanut butter, but preferably both. I also loved carbs—I would devour all the bread I could get my hands on, slathered in salted butter or dipped in olive oil and balsamic vinegar. At the dinner table, as my parents attempted to get me to eat roasted vegetables and my mom's chicken piccata, I would claim to be full after a few bites and then ask for dessert. "If you're full, how can you eat dessert?" they would ask.

"I have *three* stomach compartments," I'd confidently respond. "One for bread, one for 'real food,' and one for dessert. That compartment is still empty."

My adoration of sweets and carbs didn't waver as I grew older. I was content to eat my weight in all things carby and sweet: grilled cheese sandwiches, mac and cheese, chocolate cake, peanut butter cups, and *all* of the holiday cookies and magic cookie bars that my mom and I would spend hours in the kitchen making every December. I would even sneak out to the freezer in the garage and steal a few cookies and bars to demolish without anyone knowing.

I stayed small, never gaining too much weight despite my less-than-desirable eating habits, most likely thanks to daily workouts at cheer practice. But I struggled with debilitating headaches. At least a few times a week when I was in elementary school, I would run to the nurse with incredible migraines, unable to concentrate on my work, just wanting to go home, curl up in the dark, and go to sleep, wishing them away by the time I woke up.

My parents, divorced by then, teamed up to take me to doctor after doctor for allergy tests and CAT scans, anything to figure out what was causing the debilitating headaches. My veins were particularly hard to find, so my parents had to help the doctors hold me down so I didn't thrash around as they stuck needles in my arm, trying to draw blood. Over the years, not one test came back with *anything*. No one ever mentioned it could be related to my diet.

Fast-forward to my junior year of high school. For lunch I would go to Rubio's Coastal Grill nearly every day for a quesadilla kids meal, complete with tortilla chips and a churro, and then snack on instant ramen after school. Not much in my diet had changed since elementary school. I also began having issues with many of my longtime friendships because more and more of my friends started drinking and partying, but I was completely uninterested. My once-bubbly personality faltered, and I began to struggle with all-consuming depression and anxiety.

At this time, I also fell madly in love with baking and the process of recipe testing. I began spending a lot more time at home, in the kitchen with the KitchenAid mixer I had begged my parents to get me for my sixteenth birthday. As I worked making chocolate cake batters and sugar cookies, or experimenting with different types of pies, the social problems I faced at school seemed to fade into the background, and I could focus fully on the ingredients in front of me.

Baking was my one escape from the negative emotions I was dealing with, the thing that brought me a sense of peace and tranquility. I began seeing a therapist and taking medication, and even though, over time, I gradually started feeling better, the baking never ceased. My older sister, Shaina, saw how it lifted me up and how much I enjoyed experimenting in the kitchen. An avid food blog reader, one day she asked, "Why don't you start your own food blog?" With these words, she changed my life.

I don't think I had ever read a blog before I started my own, other than the occasional recipe post my sister would send me from some of her favorites. I launched *RachBakes* on Tumblr at the end of my junior year; it was 2010, I was sixteen, and not many people around me had heard of a food blog. I never expected *anyone* to ever look at it, but I quickly fell in love with blogging because it allowed me to meld my favorite creative outlet—baking—with writing, one of my other favorite activities. I posted recipes for decadent seven-layer rainbow cakes, brownies studded with chocolate candy bars, and twists on some of my most well-loved recipes from my favorite cookbooks. I wrote about the football games I cheered at and the colleges I was thinking about applying to. I also discovered a new hobby: photography. I was *terrible* at it in those early days, using my pixelated flip phone to take food photos under our florescent kitchen lights.

One day during the summer before my senior year of high school, a tech-wiz family friend was visiting at my dad's house. The subject of my blog came up,

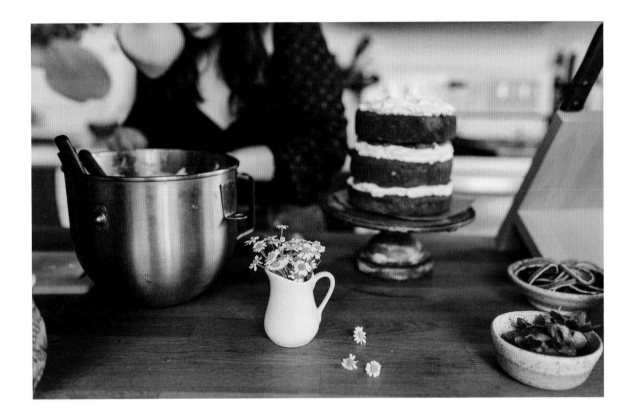

and he chuckled when he heard it was on Tumblr. "You need a *domain*," he said. I didn't know what that meant, so he walked me through it and told me to come up with a permanent website name, since RachBakes.com was already taken. After days of brainstorming with my mom, dad, sister, and anyone else around, someone suggested, "How about Crumbelina?" Taken. "Bakerina?" Taken. "Bakerita?" Available, and we all loved it. The name married my love of baking with a little bit of my Latin American heritage—the suffix *ita* in Spanish means "small," and at 5'0" tall, I am definitely that. *Bakerita* was born.

Throughout my senior year of high school, I continued baking and posting my recipes with their subpar photos, and when I started to look at colleges, one of my first questions was always: "Do the dorms have a kitchen *with an oven*?" The thought of not posting on *Bakerita* while I was at college never crossed my mind. Even as I suffered a debilitating reaction to going off antidepressants during my senior year of high school, my blog remained my place to escape. Having *Bakerita* as an outlet pulled me up during that incredibly difficult time, and it motivated me to find ways to treat my depression without medication.

Around that time, my sister, Shaina, started experiencing severe stomach pains and digestion issues. After consulting with dozens of doctors and naturopaths, she decided to cut gluten out of her diet. This was 2011, and gluten-free foods were not prevalent like they are now. Most people didn't even know what "gluten-free" meant. Eating gluten-free was especially difficult since she was living in a college dorm and limited to what was available at the dining hall, which meant the salad bar was usually her only option. Whenever she made the two-hour trip home, she would beg me to make her gluten-free treats.

This change in diet made her much more health conscious in general, and she would sit on the counter watching me as I baked. "Are you really going to put *that* much sugar in there?" "Do you really need to add so much butter?" During those moments, she was the most annoying person ever. Didn't she know that you *needed* sugar and butter to make baked goods delicious?!

Still, she was my sister, so for Shaina I began to experiment with gluten-free baking. I quickly realized I hated the seemingly bizarre gluten-free flours—like brown rice flour and garbanzo bean flour—that most recipes called for. Using them in cookie and cake recipes resulted in odd and mealy textures, and their flavors did *not* belong in my baked goods. Most recipes also included gums with names that I couldn't pronounce, and I didn't want to put these chemically sounding things into my sister's healthier treats. So I continued to experiment and turned to flours, such as oat and almond, whose flavors I already liked.

As I delved into gluten-free baking, I fell in love with the challenge of creating something that tasted decadent but was free from the allergens that caused my sister's inflammation. I was further inspired when my dad went gluten-free a year after my sister had, because now some of my main recipe tasters couldn't eat the treats I made with regular wheat flour. I continued making gluten- and sugar-filled treats for my friends at my small liberal arts college, the University of Puget Sound, but whenever I was at home in San Diego, I only baked gluten-free. I kept up that balancing act on my blog, posting both gluten-free and gluten-filled recipes, straddling both niches while not diving fully into either one.

Then, soon after graduating from college, my sister got sick. After months of doctor's appointments and tests, she discovered that she had Lyme disease:

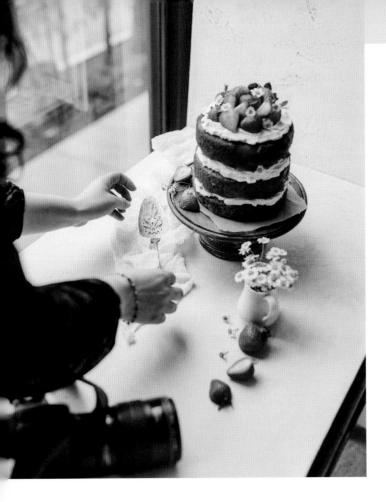

a tick-borne bacterial illness that causes fatigue, headaches, rashes, and so much more. If left untreated, it can become chronic. Shaina, the health nut that she is, became determined to cure it holistically (though she did run a few courses of antibiotics, the only way insurance companies will help treat Lyme). One way she did that was through food, attempting to starve the Lyme bacteria out of her system. That meant cutting out dairy and sugar along with the gluten she had already eliminated. To help make the transition to her new diet a little easier, she turned to me to see if there was *anything* I could bake for her.

At first I was skeptical; baking without gluten, sugar, *or* dairy? I honestly wasn't sure it was possible. With some research I discovered Paleo and vegan baking, and natural fruit sweeteners like bananas and dates. I realized that dairy-free milks, like almond and oat, could replicate dairy milks; coconut milk could replace heavy cream; and coconut oil worked well in place of butter. By trying to help Shaina cope with her disease, a whole new world of baking opened up for me. I started making her Paleo banana breads sweetened *only* with bananas, and barely sweetened Paleo granolas that were free of the oats that caused her inflammation.

Slowly but surely, my gluten-free baking transitioned into Paleo-style baking (which is free of gluten, dairy, and refined sugars), with frequent vegan baking experiments. I shared all of these recipes online and soon discovered my sister was far from alone. There was, and is, a huge community of people out there struggling with autoimmune disorders and gut issues, or simply trying to live a more healthful life, and they were searching for recipes that would taste delicious without causing inflammation in their bodies.

As soon as I graduated from college, I stopped baking with gluten entirely and finally committed to eating a fully gluten-free diet myself. The change I felt in my body was wild: much less bloating and discomfort after meals, more energy, and my debilitating headaches, which I had been getting multiple times a week since elementary school, almost entirely disappeared. My mood improved as well, and I found that the anxiety and depression I had struggled with for much of my life didn't occur nearly as often. Being my own guinea pig is what I needed to truly understand the benefits of living gluten-free.

I moved back to San Diego in 2016 and was living with my dad while looking for my own place. We decided to do a Whole30 elimination diet together as a way to reset our diets, and to give our sweet tooths a break. It was a hard four weeks for me as a baker because *no* sweeteners or desserts are allowed, but I delved headfirst into cooking, experimenting with Whole30-approved meals all month long. Along the way, I discovered even more alternatives to grains, dairy, and sugary-sweet desserts.

When we finished that Whole30 and started reincorporating different foods, it became clear that dairy was not a friend to either of us. The first night we ate cheese again our stomachs growled in protest; a reintroduction of refined sugars also didn't make us feel very good. So I cut out all dairy and refined sweeteners, and it was then that all of my recipes for *Bakerita* started following the dietary guidelines I still follow today, which are the guidelines for all the recipes in this book: **gluten-free, dairy-free, and refined sugar–free.**

When I started my blog when I was sixteen, this 180-degree change in how I bake would have been unimaginable to me. Back then, I was so resistant to healthy eating, insisting to Shaina that nothing could be as delicious as my rich chocolate brownies and cookie-dough cakes. What I didn't consider at that time was how I felt: lethargic, bloated, and unhappy.

I still remember those feelings and the resistance to changing my diet even though I knew it was for the better. There is comfort in gluten, sugar, and dairy. It's the way society tells us to eat, with big signs leading us toward fast-food places and highlighting the "convenient" yet wildly innutritious options for us in the grocery store. It becomes an act of rebellion to eat healthily: We must forge our way through restaurants, ask questions about what goes into food, be "that person." There is no shame in it, though, only self-empowerment in knowing that you're doing what's best for yourself. Eating healthily should be a source of pride, not embarrassment. Food is so much more than just nourishment for our bodies—it has an incredible impact on our mind, body, and spirit. When we realize that and shift our diet accordingly, it can lift us up in every way.

What we really need is a shift in our society, to decide that *every* person deserves to eat healthfully. This is something I am very passionate about, and I know this will never happen if the alternative to the unhealthy option isn't as delicious, easy, or convenient. My goal with each recipe in this book is to make you sigh with delight at its tastiness while leaving you feeling energized enough to go for a long walk after. These treats are still desserts, but they're nutritious, filling, and made with love.

I wrote this book because I want you to know that eating dessert is a delicious—and healthy—part of life. It doesn't need to be full of empty calories, or leave you feeling guilty, or like a blob on the couch. Dessert should bring joy, and baking should be a process of love, intention, and creativity, just like writing this book was for me. And trust me, people who don't eat a gluten-, dairy-, and refined sugar–free diet will enjoy these recipes just as much as the more traditional version. That was my intention with every recipe in this book: make it as good as the original, because eating healthy doesn't mean giving up taste.

I hope your copy of this book gets dirty with smudges of coconut oil and cacao powder, and soon has a worn spine and dog-eared pages. I hope you flip through it to find a recipe for your child's birthday cake (I recommend Shaina's Birthday Cake, page 69) or celebratory cookies. My family was a huge part of my inspiration in writing this cookbook, and I hope this book becomes a part of your family in a similar way. Whether you've been gluten- and dairy-free for years, or you've never made a gluten-free recipe in your life, I'm confident that you'll find recipes that you'll love and that will find a place on your table. They all have a special place in my heart, and I hope that they find a special place in yours too.

Introduction

DEFINING THE DIETS

Every recipe in this book is gluten-free, dairy-free, and refined sugar–free, and many of the recipes also fit into stricter dietary categories like vegan, Paleo, and grain-free. Here, I'll define each of the dietary categories that are referred to in this book.

GLUTEN-FREE: Gluten is a protein that's found in grains like wheat, rye, and barley. It helps hold things together, like glue. When you knead bread dough and it becomes elastic, that is the gluten being developed—it tends to make doughs easier to work with. However, it can be very inflammatory in many people's digestive systems. Levels of sensitivity vary widely, from slight inflammation to Celiac disease, an autoimmune disorder that leads to damage in the small intestine when gluten is consumed. Every recipe in this book is gluten-free, making them safe for people with any level of sensitivity. I replace the wheat flours traditionally found in baked goods with gluten-free flours, all listed in the following pantry section. To re-create the light and fluffy texture of wheat flour, sometimes one, two, or three different flours are necessary for the best texture.

DAIRY-FREE: Dairy refers to any products that are made out of or derived from milk from mammals, such as butter, milk, cream, cheese, yogurt, sour cream, whey, and more. Many people have a sensitivity, intolerance, or allergy to dairy. Lactose intolerance is a very common form of dairy intolerance where your body doesn't produce lactase, the enzyme needed to digest lactose, which is the sugar in milk. It causes discomfort, but is not as dangerous as a dairy allergy, which causes an allergic reaction in your body that can be deadly for those with a serious allergy. Every recipe in this book is dairy-free, except for a

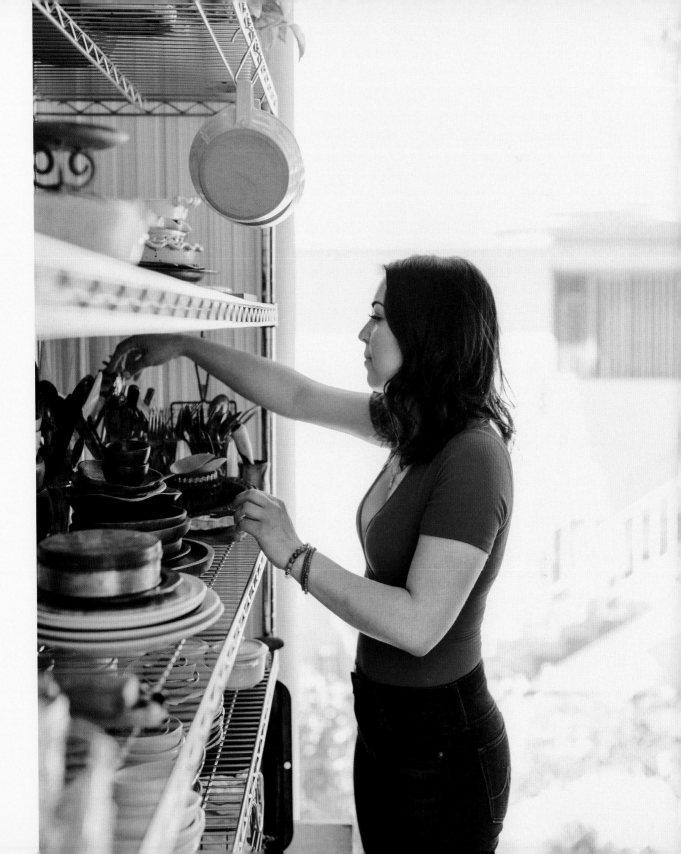

few recipes that call for ghee as an option. Ghee, which is butter that has been heated and had the dairy solids strained out of it, is a lactose-free oil. It has the flavor of butter but doesn't aggravate the digestive system of people who are lactose-intolerant (like me). If you're allergic to dairy or are vegan, use refined coconut oil or vegan butter instead. I provide a substitute in recipes where ghee is an option.

REFINED SUGAR-FREE: In this book, I don't use any refined sugars, which include white sugar (which has been bleached and stripped of any nutritional value), brown sugar, and corn syrup. In their place, I use sweeteners like coconut sugar (which is derived from coconut sap), pure maple syrup, and honey. These products are more natural and unprocessed, and therefore retain more vitamins and minerals. I don't recommend substituting a liquid sweetener for a granular sweetener in any recipe, such as substituting honey for coconut sugar, or vice versa, because it will affect the texture of the final baked good. You can, however, substitute maple syrup for honey and vice versa, though the flavor will be affected.

VEGAN: When a recipe is labeled vegan, that means it is entirely free of animal products. That means there is no dairy, eggs, or honey, which are allowed when something is simply vegetarian. Many of the recipes in this book are vegan or can be made vegan. A few recipes call for either ghee or honey, neither of which are vegan, but I include vegan options to use instead.

PALEO: The Paleo diet, sometimes referred to as the caveman diet, is free from grains (like oats and rice), beans, legumes (including peanut butter), dairy (except ghee), and refined sugars. Since all of the recipes in this book are dairy-free and refined sugar-free, only the recipes with oats, oat flour, crispy rice cereal, and peanut butter will not be Paleo-friendly.

GRAIN-FREE: This means a recipe is free from all grains: both grains that contain gluten (like wheat and barley) and gluten-free grains (like oats and rice) alike. Any grain-free recipes are inherently gluten-free, but not all gluten-free products or recipes are grain-free.

SOY-FREE: Every recipe in this book is soy-free, which is a common allergen for many people. Soy products include tofu, soy sauce, soy milk, miso, and common food additives like soy lecithin.

HOW TO STOCK YOUR KITCHEN

IN THE CABINET

GLUTEN-FREE FLOURS

I don't like store-bought gluten-free flour mixes because brands can vary so widely. My recipes call for one or two different flours—a maximum of three—to create the best texture. I keep five main flours on hand all the time, and they are the only ones called for in the book.

BUYING IN BULK

Because they're made of real, whole foods, many of the ingredients used in this book can get expensive. To drive down the costs, I prefer to buy in bulk from online retailers such as Amazon or at warehouse stores like Costco and look for the largest sizes I can find. If you bake frequently, I recommend you do so as well! Store nuts and flours in the refrigerator or freezer to help keep them fresh for an extended period of time.

BLANCHED ALMOND FLOUR: This is not the same as almond meal and will not perform the same way in recipes. Blanched almond flour is finer, whereas almond meal is not as finely ground and often includes the almond skins. Please always use blanched almond flour for the recipes in this book to get the right result.

COCONUT FLOUR: Coconut flour is unique in that it is *much* more absorbent than other flours, about three times as absorbent, usually. This means that recipes using coconut flour will generally call for a much smaller amount of flour than you're used to with more traditional flours. I do not recommend substituting any other flour for coconut flour.

TAPIOCA AND ARROWROOT STARCH: I use these often in my recipes to create a light, fluffy texture in breads and cakes, and a crispier texture in cookies. Sometimes called tapioca flour and arrowroot flour, they can generally be used interchangeably, but they do create slightly different textures, so there is a reason I call for one or the other in a recipe. I recommend having both on hand.

GLUTEN-FREE OAT FLOUR: Oat flour is simply made of ground oats. You can make it yourself by grinding oats in a blender for about 30 seconds, until floury. Make sure to seek out a gluten-free oat flour or oats, since some oats are processed in a facility that also processes gluten, which can cause cross-contamination.

SWEETENERS

COCONUT SUGAR: Coconut sugar is my go-to granulated sweetener. It's made from the sap of the flower buds of the coconut palm tree. I buy it in bulk bags from Amazon, but it's also available at Trader Joe's, Whole Foods, and many other mainstream grocery stores.

HONEY: I prefer to use raw, mild-flavored honey, but any honey will work. Keep in mind that honey is not vegan, but in most cases you can use maple syrup in its place to keep a recipe vegan.

PURE MAPLE SYRUP: Since pure maple syrup can be expensive, I buy it in big 32-ounce bottles to bring the cost down. I love maple syrup as a sweetener because it contains lots of vitamins and minerals and, of course, for its delicious flavor! Make sure you're buying pure maple syrup and not a maple-flavored syrup, which is usually made up of corn syrup and artificial colors and flavors.

STAPLES

COCONUT OIL: Coconut oil is one of my favorite and most used fats in this book. I find it to be a great replacement for butter because of the similar texture and the fact that they're both solid at cool room temperature. Because of this, coconut oil is perfect for using in cookies and other recipes where the fat needs to be whipped with the sugar. I like to keep both refined and virgin coconut oil on hand. In certain recipes, I'll call for refined coconut oil, which has had the coconut flavor removed but still retains all of the other qualities of coconut oil. This is best used in places where you want no coconut flavor to come through. If you're sensitive to coconut flavor, you can use refined coconut oil in any recipe that calls for coconut oil. Otherwise, they can be used interchangeably. In cooler climates or in a cool kitchen, coconut oil will firm up to a hard consistency. When it is warmer in your kitchen, the consistency will either be similar to softened butter or melted, depending on how warm it is. Depending on the recipe and what state your coconut oil is in, you may need to either chill, soften, or melt the coconut oil. To soften, microwave it for 10 to 15 seconds and stir until it reaches the consistency of softened butter. Melting is easy to do in the microwave, for about 30 seconds for most amounts.

COCONUT BUTTER: Coconut butter is *different* from coconut oil. Coconut oil is thinner when melted, since it's just the oil. Coconut butter, on the other hand, is the butter that comes from grinding dried coconut meat. You can make it yourself with dried unsweetened coconut (page 265). When melted, it is thick and creamy—it provides structure in a way that coconut oil does not. For that reason, one cannot be substituted for the other, unless otherwise stated. You can usually find it near the nut butters in the grocery store.

HOW TO ROAST NUTS

Toasted nuts are my favorite and can add so much flavor to a recipe. To toast nuts, I bake them at 350°F for 8 to 10 minutes, or until fragrant and golden brown in color. From time to time, I toast nuts in a skillet. The method is described in the recipes where I use a skillet. When a recipe calls for roasted or toasted nuts, use either method (in the oven or in a skillet). Either way, it's best to let them cool completely before using.

NUT BUTTERS: I love nut butter and use it in so many recipes. It works as a fat to add protein, helps keep things tender, and is so delicious. Make sure the nut and seed butters that you use are oil- and sugar-free. The only ingredients should be nuts and maybe salt. I like to keep peanut butter, almond butter, and cashew butter on hand always. I also call for sunflower seed butter and pecan butter in this book. Store these in the fridge if you don't go through them quickly. Also, since we're using natural nut butters without any emulsifiers, you'll have to make sure your nut butters are well-stirred before using.

BAKING POWDER AND BAKING SODA: If you follow a strictly grain-free diet, purchase a corn-free baking powder, like Pamela's brand. Make sure these are fresh, or they won't be as effective!

NUTS: I always have a full stock of nuts on hand because I use them so often. I like to have *lots* of cashews on hand, along with peanuts, pecans, and almonds. I buy them all raw, except peanuts. Store in the refrigerator or freezer if you don't use them quickly.

CHOCOLATE CHIPS AND CHUNKS: Chocolate can be one of the more difficult things to find in both dairy-free and refined sugar–free form. I use coconut sugar–sweetened chocolate chips from Santa Barbara Chocolate or Hu Kitchen in all of my recipes, except for when I call for chopped chocolate chunks. In that case, seek out any bars of chocolate that are coconut sugar–sweetened, such as Hu Kitchen or Eating Evolved brands, or if you're okay with some refined sugars, use a cane sugar–sweetened bar. Avoid chocolate with added stabilizers, waxes, dairy, or preservatives. Dark chocolate is nothing more exotic than bittersweet or semisweet chocolate; it's chocolate without milk solids or a lot of sugar. I refer to dark chocolate as "bittersweet chocolate" in these recipes. You may also see chocolate labeled with percentages, such as 60% cacao. This refers to the amount of cacao in the chocolate compared to the amount of sugar; therefore, a 60% chocolate bar would be 60% cacao and 40% sugar. In my recipes, I like to use anywhere between 60 and 80% cacao, but depending on how sweet or bitter you like your chocolate, you can use whatever you prefer.

SOAKING CASHEWS

A lot of my cashew-based cheesecakes and frostings call for soaked raw cashews. I find cashews blend up best after being soaked in filtered water for a minimum of 4 hours or, even better, overnight. If I'm soaking for only 4 to 6 hours, room temperature is fine. Any longer than that, I put them in the refrigerator. I don't let them soak for longer than 12 hours, or else they get mealy. When you're ready to use, drain the cashews and rinse with cool water. In a pinch, you can pour boiling water over the cashews and let them sit at room temperature for about an hour. The final product won't be quite as smooth as cashews soaked for longer, but it will do the trick!

CACAO POWDER (AND CACAO VS. COCOA): The difference between cacao and cocoa is pretty simple: In cacao products, the cacao bean has remained raw, whereas in cocoa products, the cacao bean has been roasted.

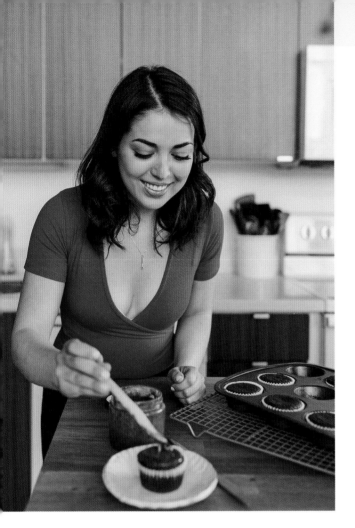

I prefer to use cacao products (cacao powder, cacao butter, and cacao nibs) over cocoa products, because cacao is packed with antioxidants, vitamins, and minerals. However, cocoa products are generally much cheaper than cacao and can be used in place of cacao in most recipes, including all of the ones in this book.

CACAO BUTTER (OR COCOA BUTTER): Cacao butter has a chocolatey flavor, but with the deep, dark flavor of the cacao powder removed. It is used in many of the white chocolate desserts, as well as many no-bake desserts. Coconut oil can usually be substituted for cacao butter if you can't get your hands on it, but the flavor will not be the same and it will have a lower melting point.

FULL-FAT COCONUT MILK: I try to use coconut milk that doesn't have gums in it. Coconut milk is sold in cartons and cans. I like to use canned coconut milk because of its texture. When you open the can, the top of the milk will usually be solid. Sir it into the can to mix with the liquid milk below or empty the contents of the can into a bowl and stir the milk until it's well combined and creamy.

COCONUT CREAM: I love whipped coconut cream as a garnish for tarts, pies, and cakes. Coconut cream is the thick, fattier part of coconut milk. When you refrigerate a can of full-fat coconut milk overnight, the cream will separate into a firm, creamy white layer on top. That's the part you want when coconut cream is called for! You can also find coconut cream by itself in 5.4-ounce or 13.5-ounce can. This will almost always be chilled when used in recipes, and you'll want to make sure it's refrigerated overnight and drained of any water at the bottom of the can before use. The Nature's Charm brand makes a great product called coconut whipping cream that whips up perfectly for garnishing—it's lightly sweetened with coconut sugar. If you can find it, I recommend using this wherever I call for whipped coconut cream.

DAIRY-FREE MILK: I always have cartons of dairy-free milks in the fridge, whether it's almond milk, cashew milk, or oat milk. These can generally be used interchangeably in recipes, just do not substitute them for full-fat coconut milk.

ROLLED OATS: Oats are naturally gluten-free, but many times are processed in facilities that also process wheat, so make sure your oats are certified gluten-free.

EXTRA-VIRGIN OLIVE OIL: I use olive oil in a few cake recipes. Make sure yours has a nice light and fruity flavor and isn't bitter at all.

FREEZE-DRIED FRUIT: I use freeze-dried strawberries and bananas to flavor some desserts. I get them from Trader Joe's, but they are also available online or in other grocery stores.

SPICES

- Sea salt
- Cinnamon
- Nutmeg
- Allspice
- Ginger

VANILLA BEAN POWDER: I use this a lot to create a bold vanilla flavor without needing to use a whole vanilla bean, which is very expensive. Vanilla bean powder is made from the entire ground pod, so it's more affordable but still very rich in flavor. A little goes a long way—I used one small jar for *all* the testing in this book. I usually can't find vanilla bean powder in stores, so I typically purchase it through Amazon. If you don't have it and don't want to buy it, you can get away with substituting two times the amount of vanilla extract, but note that you won't get the vanilla bean flecks like you do with the powder.

PURE VANILLA EXTRACT: Make sure to buy *pure* vanilla extract, and not a baker's extract, which has been diluted and has artificial "vanilla flavor" added to it.

FLAX EGGS

I use ground flax seed "eggs" as an egg replacement in many recipes in this book to keep things vegan! See below for more on grinding flax seed.

To prepare a flax egg for a recipe, combine 1 tablespoon ground flax seed with 2½ tablespoons water. Whisk together and let set for 5 to 10 minutes, or until it becomes a sticky gel texture.

Sometimes a recipe will call for 1½ or 2 flax eggs. For 1½ flax eggs, the amounts are 1 tablespoon + 1½ teaspoons ground flax seed with ¼ cup water. For 2 flax eggs, use 2 tablespoons ground flax seed with 5 tablespoons water.

FLAKY SEA SALT: I use this often to garnish the top of baked treats, particularly chocolate ones! It adds a bit of crunch and doesn't make things taste overly salty. Maldon and Jacobsen Salt Co. are my favorite brands.

IN THE REFRIGERATOR

EGGS: When I do use eggs, I make sure to buy organic and, if possible, pasture-raised. I like Vital Farms eggs from the supermarket, or getting eggs from the farmers' market when I can. I always use large eggs.

GROUND FLAX SEED: I use ground flax seed (flax meal) frequently to make flax eggs. While you can buy ground flax meal, I prefer to grind flax seed myself in my Vitamix—you can also use a clean, dry spice grinder. I do a big batch at a time and store it in an airtight jar in my fridge to keep it as fresh as possible.

EQUIPMENT

The following list details the equipment that I use to make all of the recipes in this book. Some pan sizes may seem smaller than traditionally used (like the 6-inch springform pan), but because many of the recipes are very rich and filling, a smaller dessert goes a long way. If you find yourself wanting to make a recipe that you don't have the equipment for, you can double or triple recipe quantities as needed to fit into the pans you have. I always use metal pans and recommend you do as well. Glass or ceramic pans take longer to heat and may require a longer bake time than called for.

- 6-inch springform pan
- 6-inch cake pans
- 8-inch square baking pan
- 8½ x 4½-inch loaf pan
- 8- to 9-inch round casserole-style pan
- 6½-inch cast-iron skillet
- 9-inch tart pan with removable bottom
- Donut pan
- Muffin pan
- 8- or 9-inch Bundt pan

COOKIE SCOOPS: For all the drop cookies in this book, I use the medium cookie scoop from OXO, which holds 1½ tablespoons of dough and yields a cookie that's about 2½ to 3 inches across. I also use the other two sizes of the OXO cookie scoop: The small, which holds 2 teaspoons, is great for Chocolate Chip Cookie Dough Bites (page 243) and truffles, and the large size is great for doling out batter for muffins and cupcakes.

HIGH-SPEED BLENDER: I use the Vitamix Explorian blender for all of the recipes that call for a high-powered blender or food processor.

ELECTRIC MIXER: I have a KitchenAid stand mixer that I use for whipping coconut cream

A NOTE ABOUT MIXING

Unless a recipe specifically calls for a stand mixer, high-powered blender, or food processor, I always mix my recipes by hand with my trusty whisk, wooden spoon, and/or scraper spatula. I simply prefer to do so, but if you prefer, most of the recipes can be made with a stand mixer or hand mixer to speed up the process. A paddle attachment will usually do the trick, unless a whisk is specifically called for.

and whipped frostings. An electric hand mixer will do a great job with these too.

KITCHEN SCALE: I use my scale to weigh most ingredients, which makes baking much more accurate (and you dirty fewer measuring cups). For best results, I highly recommend using one.

OVEN THERMOMETER: Recipes can result in an entirely different consistency if your oven is running too hot or too cold. Use an oven thermometer to check how your oven is running and adjust the temperature from there (or get it calibrated). You can also use it to test for hot spots in your oven. If you find certain areas are hotter, you'll want to rotate pans more often for even cooking.

PARCHMENT PAPER SHEETS: I use these to line pans for cookies, bars, brownies, and pretty much everything else. To fit them neatly into square baking pans, cut the parchment paper sheet into a square and then cut inward from each corner toward the center, about 4 inches. You should then be able to lay the parchment over the pan and press into the bottom to line it.

CHAPTER ONE

Breakfast and Snacks

A FEW TIPS AND TRICKS FOR SUCCESS:
When baking muffins and breads, be sure to leave the oven door closed throughout the baking process. Opening the door too early can release too much heat and cause the cake or cupcakes to sink in the center.

Many of these recipes can be made ahead of time, so that you can have a quick and easy breakfast or snack! I like storing muffins, breads, and scones in my freezer so that I can heat one up when I'm hungry. Granola, granola bars, pancakes, and oatmeal are all great stored in the refrigerator. Each recipe will have storage instructions so you can make them ahead of time.

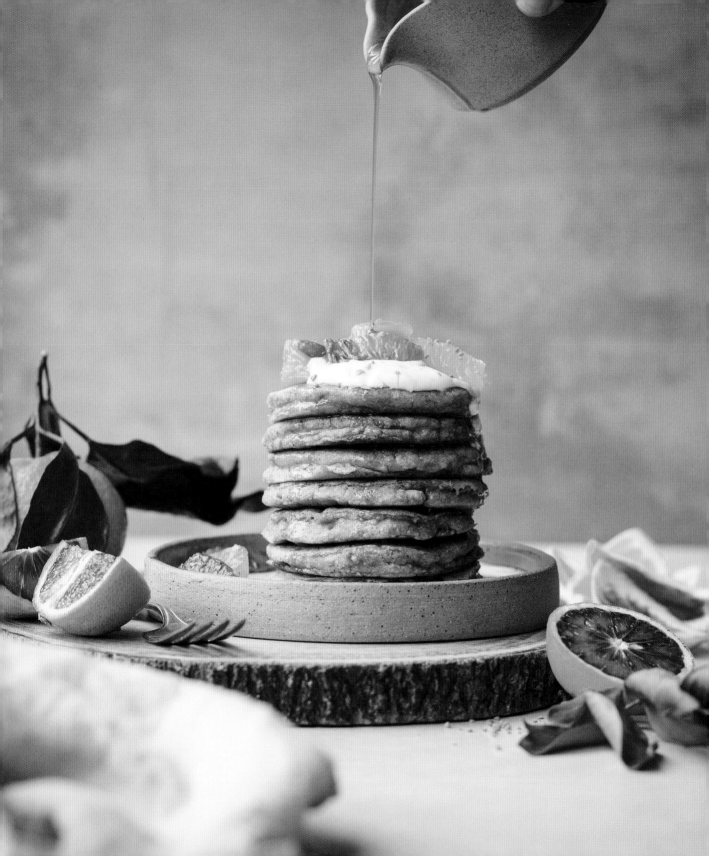

FLUFFY VEGAN PANCAKES

VEGAN • NO-BAKE • GLUTEN-FREE • DAIRY-FREE

There is nothing better than fresh pancakes on a weekend morning, and these fluffy vegan pancakes come together so quickly in the blender that you can whip them up before you've had your morning coffee. The recipe is a good starting point for making them your own too. The applesauce can be swapped out for banana or pumpkin puree to create your own flavor variations—banana-walnut or pumpkin–chocolate chip pancakes, anyone?! This recipe doubles or triples easily to serve more people.

Prep time: 15 minutes
Cook time: 15 minutes
Total time: 30 minutes
Yield: 6 to 7 small pancakes

½ cup unsweetened almond milk or other dairy-free milk

1 tablespoon apple cider vinegar

1 cup gluten-free rolled oats

¼ cup unsweetened applesauce

2 tablespoons pure maple syrup

1 teaspoon pure vanilla extract (optional)

1 tablespoon baking powder

¼ teaspoon ground cinnamon (optional)

⅛ teaspoon kosher salt

Coconut oil, for cooking

Pure maple syrup, coconut yogurt, fresh fruit, nut butter, bittersweet chocolate, or a combination of any, for serving

IN a small bowl or liquid measuring cup, combine the milk and vinegar and let the mixture stand for about 5 minutes to curdle.

IN a blender, combine the curdled milk, oats, applesauce, maple syrup, vanilla, baking powder, cinnamon if using, and salt. Blend for about 30 seconds until the oats are broken down and the batter is quite smooth. Let the batter stand for about 5 minutes to thicken up.

WHILE the batter thickens, heat a skillet or griddle pan over medium heat until it's medium-hot. Grease the pan with a small amount of coconut oil. Ladle or pour ¼ cup batter into the pan and gently spread out with the ladle or the back of a spoon. (If you're using a griddle or large pan, you can cook more than one pancake at a time.) Cook until the edges of the pancake look cooked, about 2 minutes. Flip the pancake gently and cook until golden brown, another 1 to 2 minutes. Keep the heat medium-hot to prevent burning. Transfer the pancake to a plate and keep warm by covering with a clean dish towel.

REPEAT until all of the batter is gone, adding a little more oil to the pan between each pancake and stacking them on top of each other on the plate.

SERVE warm, with maple syrup, yogurt, fresh fruit, nut butter, and/or chocolate!

IF saving these pancakes for later, wrap in plastic wrap and refrigerate for up to 4 days. Reheat in the microwave for 15 to 30 seconds.

Prep time: 10 minutes
Bake time: 20 minutes
Total time: 30 minutes
Yield: 12 muffins

∙∙∙∙∙∙∙∙∙∙∙∙∙∙∙∙∙∙∙∙∙∙∙∙∙∙∙∙∙∙∙∙∙∙∙∙∙∙∙

¾ **cup unsweetened almond milk**

1 **tablespoon apple cider vinegar**

1½ **cups (144g) blanched almond flour**

1 **cup (172g) cornmeal**

½ **cup (57g) tapioca flour**

½ **cup (72g) coconut sugar**

2 **teaspoons baking powder**

1 **teaspoon baking soda**

1¼ **teaspoons kosher salt**

¾ **teaspoon ground cinnamon**

⅓ **cup (67g) refined coconut oil, melted**

2 **flax eggs (see Tip)**

1 **cup fresh blueberries, plus more for topping if you like**

Tip

To make 2 flax eggs, mix 2 tablespoons ground flax seed with 5 tablespoons water. Whisk well and then set aside at room temperature for about 10 minutes to gel.

BLUEBERRY CORNMEAL MUFFINS

VEGAN • GLUTEN-FREE • DAIRY-FREE

Blueberry muffins are one of the greatest comfort foods. It's hard to beat the smell of sweet bubbling blueberries laced with cinnamon and sugar wafting from your oven—until you pull one out of the oven and slather it with a little butter, honey, or nut butter. This recipe is a twist on the classic favorite, thanks to the addition of cornmeal, which adds a little bit of texture to the timeless flavors. I like keeping muffins in the freezer so I can heat one up in the morning for a quick breakfast or snack.

∙∙∙

PREHEAT the oven to 375°F. Line one 12-cup or two 6-cup muffin pans with paper liners.

COMBINE the almond milk and vinegar in a bowl and let sit for about 5 minutes to allow the milk to curdle.

MEANWHILE, whisk together the almond flour, cornmeal, tapioca flour, coconut sugar, baking powder, baking soda, salt, and cinnamon in a large bowl, making sure to get all the clumps out.

ADD the melted coconut oil and flax eggs to the milk mixture and whisk together until smooth. Add the wet mixture to the dry ingredients and stir until smooth and combined. Fold in the blueberries.

DIVIDE the batter among the 12 lined muffin cups, filling each about three-quarters full. Sprinkle some extra blueberries on top of each muffin, if desired. Bake until golden brown and a toothpick inserted into the center of a muffin comes out clean, about 20 minutes.

LET the muffins cool in the pan for about 15 minutes, then remove from the pan and let cool completely on wire racks, still in the paper liners. You can also serve the muffins warm, if desired. In fact, I recommend trying one warm!

STORE in an airtight container at room temperature for up to 3 days, or in the refrigerator for up to 1 week. They can also be frozen for up to 3 months. If freezing, wrap well in plastic or beeswax wrap and then place in an airtight container to prevent freezer burn.

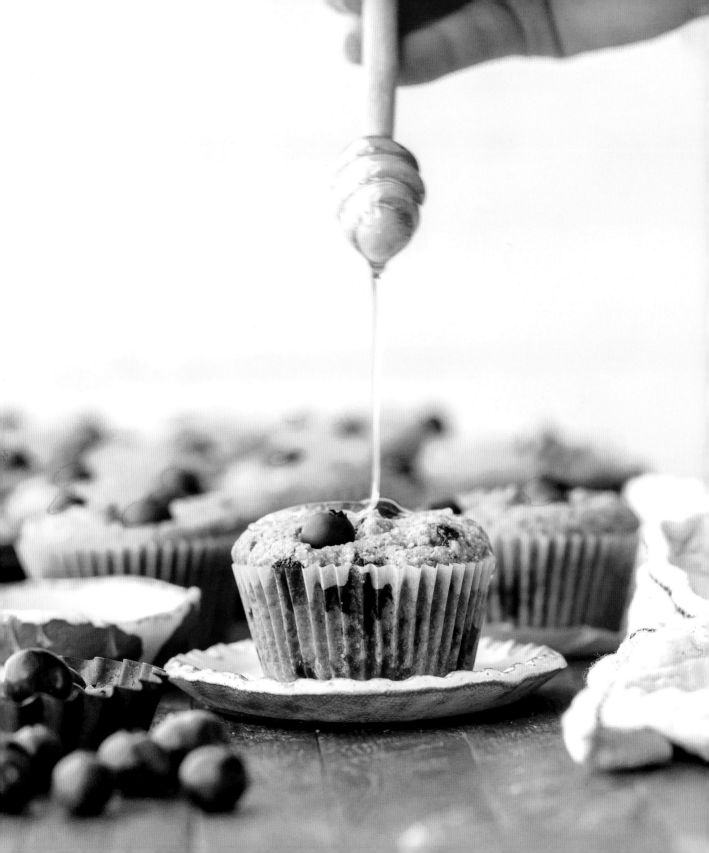

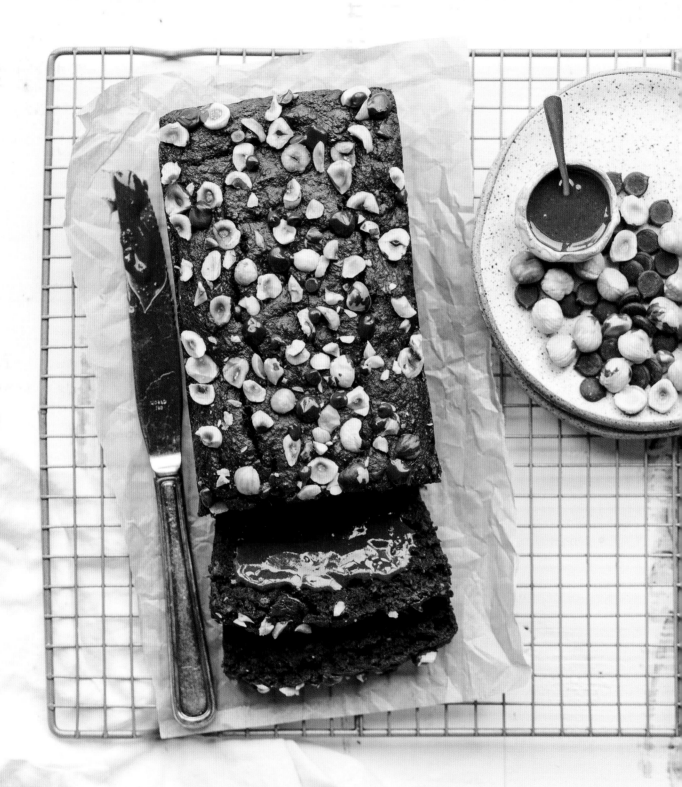

CHOCOLATE-HAZELNUT BANANA BREAD

VEGAN • GLUTEN-FREE • DAIRY-FREE

Growing up, there were few things more exciting than seeing a bunch of overripe bananas on the counter at Mom's house—that meant that banana bread was in the near future. Back in those days, we used a box mix for our banana bread, but now I rarely make the same flavor of banana bread twice. I'm always coming up with a unique take on it and experimenting with different flavors . . . but this chocolate and hazelnut version is a new favorite that broke my habit of experimentation. The bread is laced with homemade chocolate hazelnut butter and lots of ripe bananas to keep it soft and flavorful, then topped with chocolate and hazelnuts for texture—it makes the perfect breakfast or dessert.

PREHEAT the oven to 350°F. Line an 8½ × 4½-inch loaf pan with parchment paper and grease lightly with coconut oil. (You can also use a 9 × 5-inch loaf pan; the finished loaf of banana bread will be a little thinner.)

IN a large mixing bowl, combine the mashed bananas, coconut sugar, almond milk, chocolate hazelnut butter, coconut oil, and ground flax seed. Whisk well to combine. The batter should be smooth with only a few small chunks of banana.

IN a separate bowl, whisk together the hazelnut flour, oat flour, cacao powder, baking soda, baking powder, and salt. Using a rubber spatula, fold the dry ingredients into the wet ingredients and stir until well mixed. Fold in the chocolate chips.

POUR the batter into the prepared loaf pan. Top with hazelnuts or chocolate chips, or both, if using.

BAKE for 50 minutes to 1 hour, until a toothpick or knife inserted near the middle of the loaf comes out clean. If you're using a 9 × 5-inch pan, check on the bread after 40 to 45 minutes.

LET the bread cool completely in the pan before removing and slicing. Store the bread, tightly wrapped in plastic wrap or foil or in a sealed container on the counter, for up to 3 days. Refrigerate for up to 1 week or freeze for up to 6 months. I like to freeze slices that I can heat in the microwave whenever I want a slice of this bread!

Prep time: 10 minutes
Bake time: 50 minutes
Total time: 1 hour
Yield: 10 slices

- 1⅓ cups (303g) mashed overripe bananas (3 or 4 small or medium bananas)
- ⅓ cup (48g) coconut sugar
- ¼ cup unsweetened almond milk or other dairy-free milk
- ¼ cup (64g) Chocolate Hazelnut Butter (page 269)
- ¼ cup (50g) refined coconut oil, melted
- 2 tablespoons ground flax seed
- 1 cup (112g) hazelnut flour (see Tip)
- ¾ cup (90g) gluten-free oat flour
- ½ cup (42g) cacao powder
- 1 teaspoon baking soda
- 1 teaspoon baking powder
- ½ teaspoon kosher salt
- 4 ounces bittersweet chocolate chips or chopped chocolate (about ⅔ cup)
- Small handful chopped hazelnuts, for topping (optional)
- Small handful chocolate chips, for topping (optional)

Tip

You can make hazelnut flour yourself by grinding hazelnuts in a blender until finely ground and floury. Bob's Red Mill also makes it ready to purchase.

Prep time: 15 minutes
Bake time: 45 minutes
Total time: 1 hour
Yield: 8 servings (about 6 cups)

- 1½ cups (144g) gluten-free rolled oats
- 1½ cups (169g) raw pecans, roughly chopped
- 1 cup (60g) unsweetened coconut flakes
- 2 tablespoons chia seeds
- 2 tablespoons hemp seeds
- ½ cup (122g) unsweetened applesauce
- ⅓ cup (48g) coconut sugar
- ¼ cup (50g) refined coconut oil, melted
- ¼ cup (64g) creamy pecan, cashew, or (42g) almond butter
- 2 tablespoons pure maple syrup
- 1 tablespoon ground cinnamon
- 1 teaspoon pure vanilla extract
- ½ teaspoon ground nutmeg
- ¼ teaspoon ground cloves
- ¼ teaspoon allspice
- ¼ teaspoon sea salt
- ½ cup dried unsweetened apple rings, chopped

APPLE-CINNAMON GRANOLA

VEGAN • GLUTEN-FREE • DAIRY-FREE

Want to make your kitchen smell like a fall dream? Bake up a batch of apple-cinnamon granola! It brings the sweet taste of fall to your kitchen all year round, and I can't put into words how deliciously spiced it will make your kitchen smell. It's sweet and crunchy, loaded with warm spices like cinnamon, nutmeg, and allspice, and tossed with pecans and dried apple chunks for added texture. This makes a pretty big batch for just me, so I love reusing old jars to package some up and gift it—guaranteed to bring a smile to your loved ones' faces!

PREHEAT the oven to 300°F. Line a large baking sheet (about 16 × 12 inches) with parchment paper. Use two baking sheets if your sheets are small.

IN a large bowl, mix together the oats, pecans, coconut flakes, chia seeds, and hemp seeds.

IN a separate bowl, whisk together the applesauce, coconut sugar, coconut oil, nut butter, maple syrup, cinnamon, vanilla, nutmeg, cloves, allspice, and salt.

POUR the wet ingredients over the dry and stir until the dry ingredients are coated. Spread the granola mixture on the prepared baking sheet(s) and lightly press to create an even layer. It will be about ¼ inch thick.

BAKE for 45 to 55 minutes, turning the pan every 20 minutes to ensure even baking, until golden brown and dry to the touch.

LET the granola cool on the baking sheet without disturbing it. This helps the granola set so that clusters form. Once cool, toss in the chopped dried apples.

STORE in an airtight container or bag at room temperature for about 2 weeks, or in the refrigerator for up to 2 months.

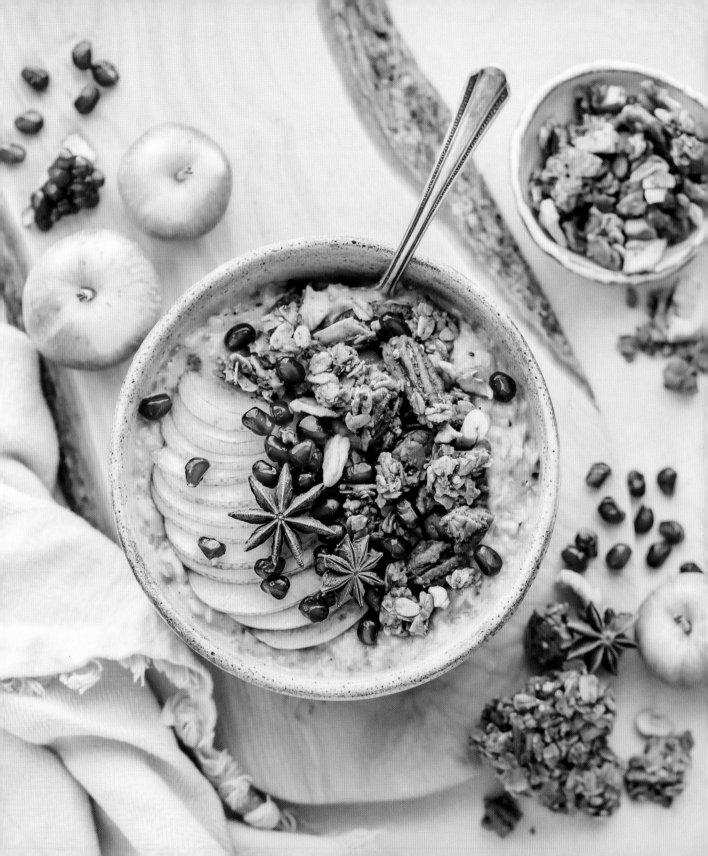

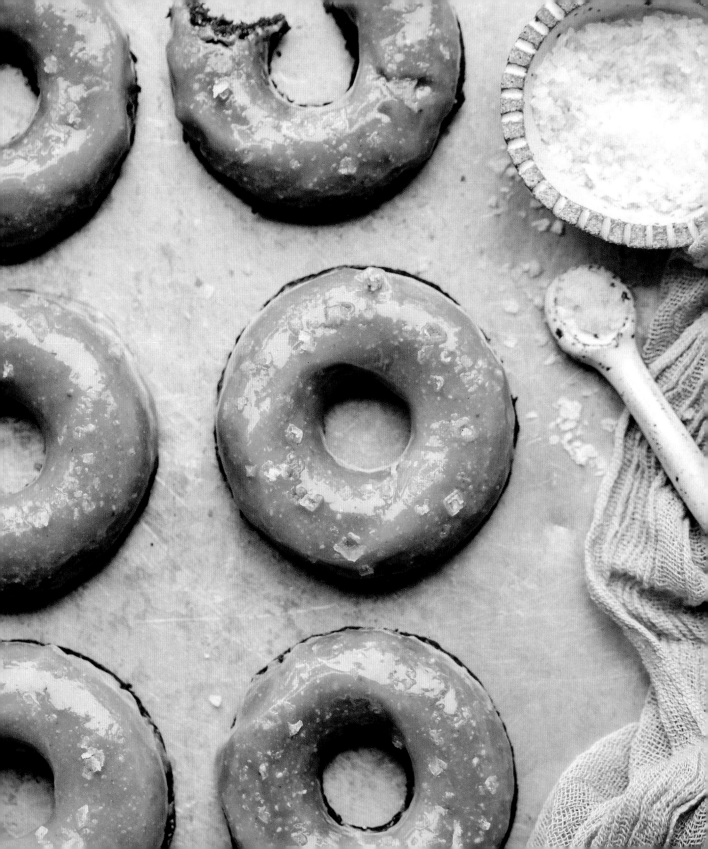

BAKED CHOCOLATE DONUTS

GRAIN-FREE • PALEO • GLUTEN-FREE • DAIRY-FREE

When I was a kid, my dad was on a mission to figure out some healthy snacks for me to eat. One day, he asked me a seemingly simple question: "What's your favorite kind of nut?" After a few moments of pondering, my six-year-old self had a light bulb moment and responded, "A donut!" In those days I tended to choose donuts that were the size of my face and coated in sugary chocolate frosting. While I'm still a big donut fan, they're just a little different these days—although I'm still partial to chocolate. These chocolate donuts are soft and cakey, with a scrumptious salted maple glaze. There is some mashed banana to add some softness and sweetness and the flavor does come through a bit, so if you're not much into banana, feel free to use unsweetened applesauce in its place.

PREHEAT the oven to 350°F; lightly grease one 12-cavity or two 6-cavity donut pans with coconut oil.

FOR THE DONUTS: In a large mixing bowl, whisk together the almond flour, tapioca flour, coconut sugar, cacao powder, baking soda, and salt.

IN a separate mixing bowl, stir the mashed banana with the milk, eggs, coconut oil, and vanilla. Stir this mixture into the dry ingredients and stir until combined.

SPOON the batter into the prepared donut pan, filling each cavity about two-thirds full. You can also pipe the batter into the cavities using a piping bag or zipped plastic bag with a corner snipped off. Bake for 10 minutes, until the donuts are firm and a toothpick inserted in a donut comes out clean. Let the donuts cool completely before carefully removing them from the pan.

FOR THE GLAZE: Combine the cashew butter, maple syrup, and coconut oil in a bowl and whisk to combine. Dip the top of each donut in the glaze and let any excess drip off, then arrange on a baking sheet. Sprinkle lightly with flaky sea salt. Refrigerate the donuts for about 1 hour or longer to let the glaze set.

STORE the donuts, tightly sealed, in the refrigerator for up to 5 days, or in the freezer for about 1 month.

Prep time: 15 minutes
Bake time: 10 minutes
Total time: 25 minutes
Yield: 12 donuts

FOR THE DONUTS
1 cup (96g) blanched almond flour

⅓ cup (38g) tapioca flour

⅔ cup (96g) coconut sugar

½ cup (48g) cacao powder

½ teaspoon baking soda

½ teaspoon kosher salt

About ½ cup mashed ripe banana (2 medium bananas)

⅓ cup dairy-free milk, such as unsweetened almond milk

2 large eggs, at room temperature

¼ cup (50g) refined coconut oil, melted

1 teaspoon pure vanilla extract

FOR THE GLAZE
¼ cup smooth cashew butter (see Tip)

2 tablespoons pure maple syrup

2 tablespoons refined coconut oil, melted and cooled

Flaky sea salt, for sprinkling

Tip

Switch out the cashew butter in the glaze for any kind of nut butter. Peanut butter would be delicious here!

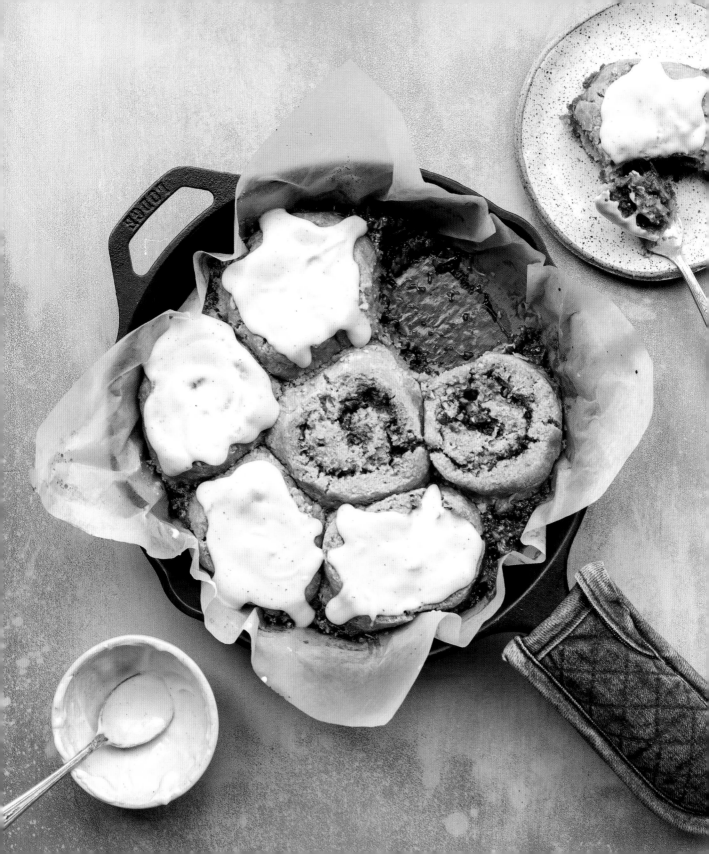

ONE-HOUR CINNAMON ROLLS

PALEO · GRAIN-FREE · VEGAN · GLUTEN-FREE · DAIRY-FREE

My sister, Shaina, has been begging me to make cinnamon rolls for her for as long as I can remember. But not just any cinnamon rolls. She avoids grains, so they had to be grain-free. I was stressed about developing a recipe that would satisfy her cravings since one could say she is a cinnamon roll aficionado—any time we're at a healthier restaurant that has a gluten-free cinnamon roll, it's on her plate. After testing this recipe a few times, though, I'd say I nailed it: When I brought them to our Christmas gathering, they not only got approval from her, but from my family members who never eat gluten-free/Paleo/vegan baked goods. They're fluffy, soft, full of cinnamon flavor, and, since they're made without yeast, ready within an hour. They also have a sticky bun–style bottom layer that's crunchy, chewy, and so decadent. Don't forget to warm them up and top them with loads of the tangy "cream cheese"–style icing for the most delicious treat!

BEFORE you begin, soak the cashews for the glaze. Put the cashews in a large bowl and add enough water to cover by 1 or 2 inches. Let the cashews soak for at least 4 hours on the countertop. If soaking for longer, refrigerate for up to 12 hours. If you don't have time for the longer soak, cover the cashews with boiling water and let them soak for 1 hour.

PREHEAT the oven to 400°F.

GREASE a 9×9-inch or 8×8-inch square baking dish with coconut oil. (It will be easier to fit 12 rolls in the larger pan than the 8×8-inch pan, which is perfect for 9 rolls. Or, a slightly larger rectangular pan, a similarly sized round casserole dish, or a cast-iron skillet will work, too.)

FOR THE SWEET PECAN BOTTOMS: Drizzle the melted ghee in the bottom of the pan. Swirl it around to cover the bottom. Sprinkle the coconut sugar evenly on top and then top with the pecans. Drizzle the honey over the pecans.

FOR THE DOUGH: Whisk together the milk and vinegar in a medium bowl and set aside for about 5 minutes to give the milk time to curdle.

Prep time: 25 minutes
Bake time: 25 minutes
Total time: 50 minutes (plus soaking the cashews)
Yield: 9 to 12 cinnamon rolls

1 cup (120g) raw cashews

FOR THE SWEET
PECAN BOTTOMS
3 tablespoons ghee or vegan butter, melted
⅓ cup (48g) coconut sugar
½ cup (57g) chopped pecans
2 tablespoons honey

FOR THE DOUGH
1 cup dairy-free milk, such as unsweetened almond milk, warmed slightly
1 tablespoon apple cider vinegar
6 tablespoons (75g) refined coconut oil, melted and cooled
2 teaspoons pure vanilla extract
3½ cups (336g) blanched almond flour
1 cup (113g) tapioca flour, plus more for rolling
¼ cup (36g) coconut sugar
2 teaspoons baking powder
½ teaspoon baking soda
¾ teaspoon kosher salt
½ teaspoon ground cinnamon
¼ cup (20g) psyllium husks

CONTINUES

FOR THE FILLING

6 tablespoons ghee or vegan butter, softened

¼ cup coconut sugar

1 tablespoon ground cinnamon

¾ cup chopped pecans (optional)

FOR THE GLAZE

½ cup canned full-fat coconut milk

¼ cup pure maple syrup

1 tablespoon fresh lemon juice

½ teaspoon apple cider vinegar

¼ teaspoon vanilla bean powder, or ½ teaspoon pure vanilla extract

Pinch of salt

Tip

Store leftover rolls in an airtight container in the fridge for up to 5 days. I like heating them up before enjoying.

ADD the melted coconut oil and vanilla to the curdled milk and whisk to combine.

IN a separate mixing bowl, whisk together the almond flour, tapioca flour, coconut sugar, baking powder, baking soda, salt, and cinnamon.

ADD the psyllium husks to the milk mixture (don't do this before this point or the liquid will become too thick), whisk it in, and then immediately add the wet ingredients to the dry. Use a spatula or wooden spoon to stir the ingredients together until a dough is formed. It will be relatively soft and just a little sticky. If it's very sticky, add 1 or 2 tablespoons additional tapioca flour.

LAY a large sheet of parchment paper or plastic wrap on a work surface and dust generously with tapioca flour. Gather up the dough and put it on the paper. Press the dough into a large rectangle; then use a rolling pin to roll the dough into an approximate 12 × 8-inch rectangle that is about ¼ inch thick.

FOR THE FILLING: In a small bowl, stir together the ghee, coconut sugar, and cinnamon. Use a small offset spatula to spread it over the dough. If using, sprinkle the pecans on top and lightly press them into the dough.

USE the parchment paper or plastic wrap to help roll the dough lengthwise into a log, keeping it as tightly rolled as possible.

WITH a serrated or very sharp knife, gently slice the log into evenly sized rolls, each 1 to 2 inches thick, to make 9 to 12 rolls. Arrange the rolls, cut-side up, in the prepared pan, positioning them so that they touch but are not crowded. Bake for 25 to 30 minutes, until golden brown.

FOR THE GLAZE: While the rolls bake, drain the cashews and rinse. Place them in a high-powered blender. Add the remaining glaze ingredients and blend on medium speed for 2 to 4 minutes, until the glaze is supersmooth and creamy. If you are not serving the rolls right away, store the glaze in an airtight jar in the refrigerator.

TO serve, drizzle the glaze over the warm rolls.

FLAKY BERRY PIE SQUARES

PALEO • GRAIN-FREE • VEGAN • GLUTEN-FREE • DAIRY-FREE

When I was in middle school, every day after my morning P.E. class I would head to the vending machines with my best friends and get myself a Pop-Tart. It was gooey, way too sweet, and I loved every bite. I've been wanting to make a healthier, homemade version for a while and it was one of the first things on my cookbook recipe brainstorm list. The result is a nostalgic treat that brings me right back to middle school—minus the stomachaches. You can use whatever berry or berry combo you like in the filling.

FOR THE BERRY FILLING: Combine the berries and maple syrup in a microwave-safe bowl and cover with plastic wrap. Microwave for 2 minutes. Mash the hot berries with a large fork, then mash in the chia seeds and lemon juice. Cover with plastic wrap and microwave for another minute, until bubbling. Transfer the filling to the refrigerator to cool while preparing the crust.

FOR THE CRUST: Combine the almond flour, tapioca flour, coconut oil, ground flax seed, coconut sugar, and salt in the bowl of a food processor fitted with the metal blade or in a mixing bowl. Pulse the processor or blend with a pastry blender until only very small bits of coconut oil remain and the mixture resembles coarse meal.

ADD the cold water and pulse or mix until the dough comes together. If you're mixing in a bowl, you may want to use your hands to bring the dough together at the end. Add additional water if needed to ensure the dough holds together in a ball.

PUT the dough on a piece of parchment paper that's been dusted with tapioca flour. Dust the top of the dough with more tapioca flour and roll into a large rectangle, about 8 × 12 inches and a little less than ¼ inch thick. To help with sticking, put another sheet of parchment paper on top of the dough and roll the rolling pin over the paper to flatten the dough.

CONTINUES

Prep time: 1 hour
Chill time: 1 hour
Bake time: 30 minutes
Total time: 2½ hours
Yield: 4 pie squares

FOR THE BERRY FILLING
2 cups fresh berries (about 1 pint), such as a mixture of strawberries, blueberries, and raspberries

2 tablespoons pure maple syrup

2 tablespoons chia seeds

1 tablespoon fresh lemon juice

FOR THE CRUST
1 cup (96g) blanched almond flour

1 cup (113g) tapioca flour, plus more for rolling out the dough

6 tablespoons (75g) refined coconut oil, softened (see Tip)

3 tablespoons ground flax seed

2 tablespoons coconut sugar

¼ teaspoon kosher salt

3 tablespoons cold water

3 to 4 tablespoons dairy-free milk, such as unsweetened almond milk; or 1 large egg, lightly beaten

FOR THE GLAZE
3 tablespoons coconut butter, plus more for drizzling (optional)

1 tablespoon refined coconut oil, softened

1 teaspoon crushed freeze-dried strawberries (2 to 3 freeze-dried strawberries)

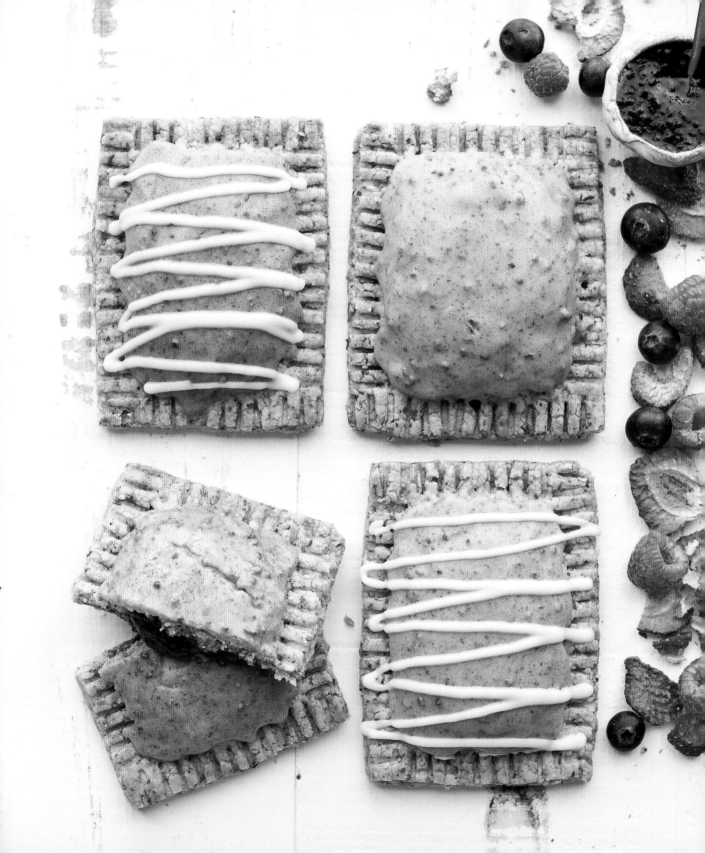

LEAVE the dough rectangle on the parchment paper and cut crosswise into four 3-inch-wide strips, then cut each strip in half crosswise for a total of eight 3 × 4-inch rectangles.

TOP four of the dough rectangles with a heaping tablespoon of the cooled filling, making sure to keep it toward the center, away from the edges. Top each with a plain dough rectangle, using a small spatula to move the dough. Use a fork to press the edges together all the way around. Carefully slide the parchment paper with the squares onto a baking sheet. Refrigerate for at least 1 hour to firm up the pastries before baking.

WHEN you're ready to bake, preheat the oven to 350°F. Use a pastry brush to brush the squares with dairy-free milk (or beaten egg, if you're not vegan). Bake for 30 minutes, until golden brown. Let cool completely before glazing.

FOR THE GLAZE: Melt the coconut butter and coconut oil in a small microwave-safe bowl in the microwave, about 30 seconds. Whisk until smooth and then whisk in the crushed freeze-dried strawberries. Spoon 1 tablespoon of the glaze over each pastry, drizzle with coconut butter, if desired, then refrigerate for at least 15 minutes to set up before serving.

STORE the glazed squares in the refrigerator for up to 3 days (they're best the first day, though), or store the unglazed squares, tightly wrapped, in the freezer for up to 3 months. Defrost the frozen squares in the toaster oven at 350°F for about 10 minutes or until warmed through.

Tip

The coconut oil should be the texture of firm chilled butter. If it melts to a liquid because the kitchen is too warm, refrigerate for 15 to 20 minutes until it solidifies.

Prep time: 2 minutes
Cook time: 8 minutes
Total time: 10 minutes
Yield: 1 serving

⅓ **cup (36g) gluten-free rolled oats**

1 **medium ripe banana, mashed**

½ **cup dairy-free milk, such as unsweetened almond milk**

BANANA-SWEETENED OATMEAL
VEGAN • NO-BAKE • GLUTEN-FREE • DAIRY-FREE

Growing up, I thought I hated oatmeal—I found it mushy, flavorless, and entirely unappetizing. Then my sister showed me how she makes her oatmeal: sweetened with a ripe banana, usually with cocoa powder added, and topped with all sorts of superfood goodies. I was a quick convert, and now I wake up craving warm, banana-sweetened oats. Over the years that I've been sharing variations on this recipe on my website, I've converted many oatmeal haters into oatmeal lovers. I took her base recipe and ran with it: I list a few favorite topping combos below, but your imagination is the limit here. I love the chocolate berry version and can never resist a healthy drizzle of nut butter on top—but see what you've got on hand and what calls to you!

IN a small saucepan, combine the oats, mashed banana, and milk. Simmer over medium heat, stirring occasionally, until the milk has been absorbed by the oats, 5 to 10 minutes. Spoon into a bowl and top with the desired topping (see Variations). Enjoy immediately!

Variations

PB&J OATMEAL: Top the oatmeal with a swirl of naturally sweetened jam and another of peanut butter or another nut butter.

CHOCOLATE-STRAWBERRY OATMEAL: Mix in 1 tablespoon unsweetened cocoa with the milk to make chocolate oatmeal. Top with ¼ cup diced strawberries and 1 tablespoon chopped bittersweet chocolate or mini chocolate chips.

ALMOND BUTTER-COCONUT OATMEAL: Mix in 1 tablespoon unsweetened cocoa with the milk to make chocolate oatmeal. Top with 1 tablespoon coconut flakes, 1 tablespoon chopped almonds, 1 tablespoon bittersweet chocolate chips, and a drizzle of almond butter, gently warmed if it's not drizzly.

PEACHES-N-CREAM OATMEAL: Top the oatmeal with diced fresh peaches and a dollop of coconut yogurt.

CHOCOLATE-PEANUT BUTTER OATMEAL: Mix in
1 tablespoon unsweetened cocoa with the milk to make chocolate
oatmeal. Top with 1 tablespoon peanuts, 1 tablespoon bittersweet
chocolate chips, and a drizzle of peanut butter, gently warmed if
it's not drizzly.

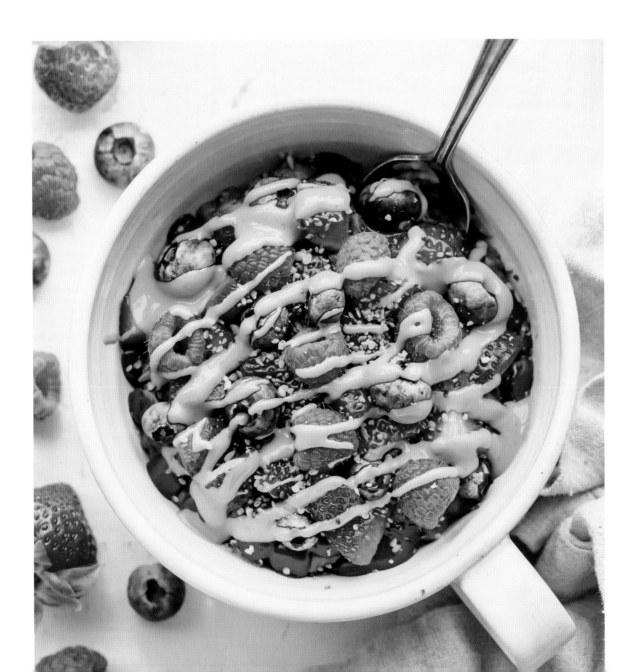

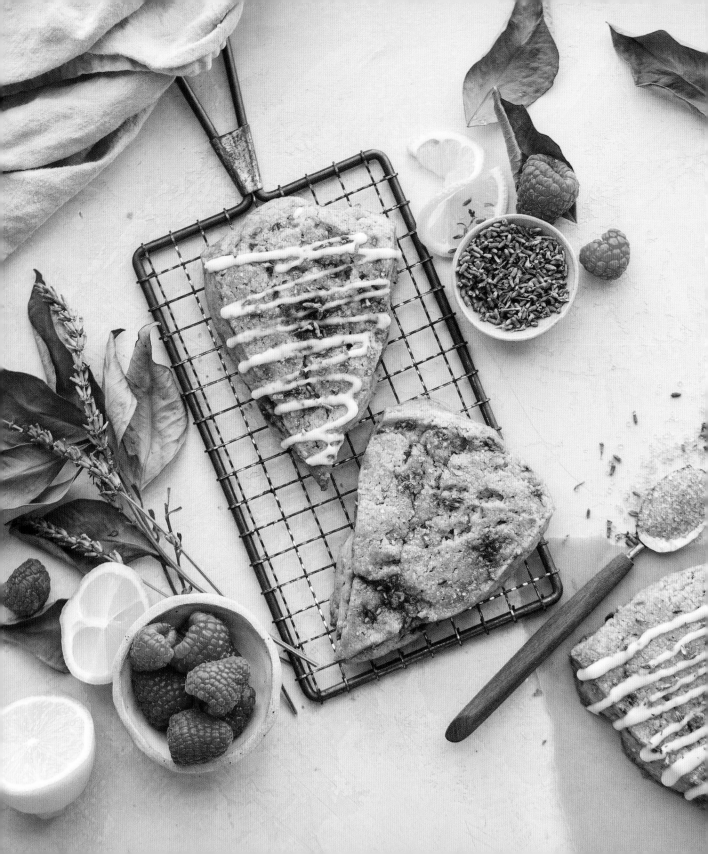

LAVENDER-LEMON RASPBERRY SCONES

PALEO • GRAIN-FREE • VEGAN • GLUTEN-FREE • DAIRY-FREE

For years, when I heard the word "scone," the words *dry*, *crumbly*, and *tasteless* came to mind. But when I studied abroad in London during my junior year of college, I had scones with tea regularly and realized what a scone could and should be: tender, flaky, and delicious. While most traditional British scones don't have mix-ins, this is my Americanized twist. The lavender adds a subtle floral note that's complemented perfectly by the tart lemon and berries. My favorite way to enjoy these scones is to reheat them in the oven and slather them with a little jam and/or vegan butter.

LINE a baking sheet with parchment paper and dust it with arrowroot starch. Rub the lavender between the palms of your hands to break it up and release its aroma.

IN the bowl of a food processor fitted with the metal blade or in a large mixing bowl, pulse or whisk the lavender, almond flour, arrowroot starch, coconut sugar, baking powder, salt, and lemon zest. Add the coconut oil and pulse or use a pastry cutter or fork to work the coconut oil into the dry ingredients until only small bits of coconut oil remain.

IN a small mixing bowl, whisk together the coconut milk, lemon juice, and flax egg. Add to the dry ingredients and pulse or stir until completely combined. Fold in the raspberries (do this by hand).

PUT the dough on the parchment paper, dust with arrowroot starch, and press into a round about 1½ inches thick and 8 inches in diameter. Refrigerate for 1 hour until chilled.

PREHEAT the oven to 375°F.

CUT the chilled round into 8 triangular scones. Separate them from each other so they don't touch and leave them on the parchment-covered baking sheet. Sprinkle with raw turbinado sugar if using. Bake for about 30 minutes, until golden brown.

SERVE warm, drizzled with coconut butter, if desired. Refrigerate in an airtight container for up to a week.

Prep time: 20 minutes
Chill time: 1 hour
Bake time: 30 minutes
Total time: 1 hour 50 minutes
Yield: 8 scones

1¼ teaspoons dried culinary-grade lavender

2¼ cups (216g) blanched almond flour

¾ cup (96g) arrowroot starch, plus more for dusting

¼ cup (36g) coconut sugar

1¼ teaspoons baking powder

½ teaspoon sea salt

Grated zest of 1 medium lemon

½ cup (100g) refined coconut oil, solid

⅓ cup canned full-fat coconut milk

2 tablespoons fresh lemon juice

1 flax egg (see Tip)

1 cup fresh raspberries

Raw turbinado sugar, for sprinkling (optional)

Coconut butter, for garnish (optional)

Tip

To make a flax egg, mix 1 tablespoon ground flax seed with 2½ tablespoons water. Stir well and then let the mixture sit for about 10 minutes to gel.

Prep time: 15 minutes
Bake time: 16 minutes
Total time: 31 minutes
Yield: 12 muffins

1 cup mashed bananas
  (2 large bananas)

3 large eggs, at room
  temperature

3 tablespoons refined coconut
  oil, melted

¼ cup dairy-free milk, such as
  unsweetened almond milk

⅓ cup (85g) creamy
  almond butter

1 teaspoon pure vanilla extract

⅓ cup (43g) coconut flour

1 teaspoon ground cinnamon

¾ teaspoon baking soda

¾ teaspoon baking powder

½ teaspoon kosher salt

½ cup freshly shredded carrot

½ cup chopped toasted pecans

⅓ cup golden raisins

Tip

To make the muffins
nut-free, simply use a
nut-free butter (like
sunflower seed butter
or tahini) and a nut-free
milk, and skip the pecans.

MORNING GLORY MUFFINS
PALEO • GRAIN-FREE • GLUTEN-FREE • DAIRY-FREE

This recipe has become a staple for so many people who follow my blog, and for good reason! These fully loaded muffins are the breakfast you've been dreaming of—they're easy to make and filled with all sorts of healthful goodness. Thanks to the bananas, shredded carrots, and almond butter, they're incredibly tender and flavorful. Toasted pecans and golden raisins add chewy and crunchy textures and can easily be swapped out for your favorite nuts and dried fruit. Between the sweetness of the ripe bananas and the raisins, there's no need for any added sugar! Your mornings will thank you!

PREHEAT the oven to 350°F. Line the 12 cups of a muffin tin with paper liners or grease with coconut oil.

IN a large mixing bowl or stand mixer fitted with the paddle attachment, mix together the mashed bananas, eggs, coconut oil, almond milk, almond butter, and vanilla until fully combined. Add the coconut flour, cinnamon, baking soda, baking powder, and salt and mix well. Fold in the shredded carrot, toasted pecans, and raisins.

DIVIDE the batter among the prepared muffin cups, filling each about two-thirds full. Bake for 16 to 19 minutes, until a toothpick inserted into the center of a muffin comes out clean and the top springs back when pressed with a fingertip.

COOL the muffin tin on a wire rack for about 10 minutes. Remove the muffins from the tin and let them cool completely on the rack.

STORE the muffins in an airtight container at room temperature for 2 days, or in the refrigerator for up to a week; or tightly wrap and freeze for up to 3 months. If frozen, microwave for about 30 seconds to thaw.

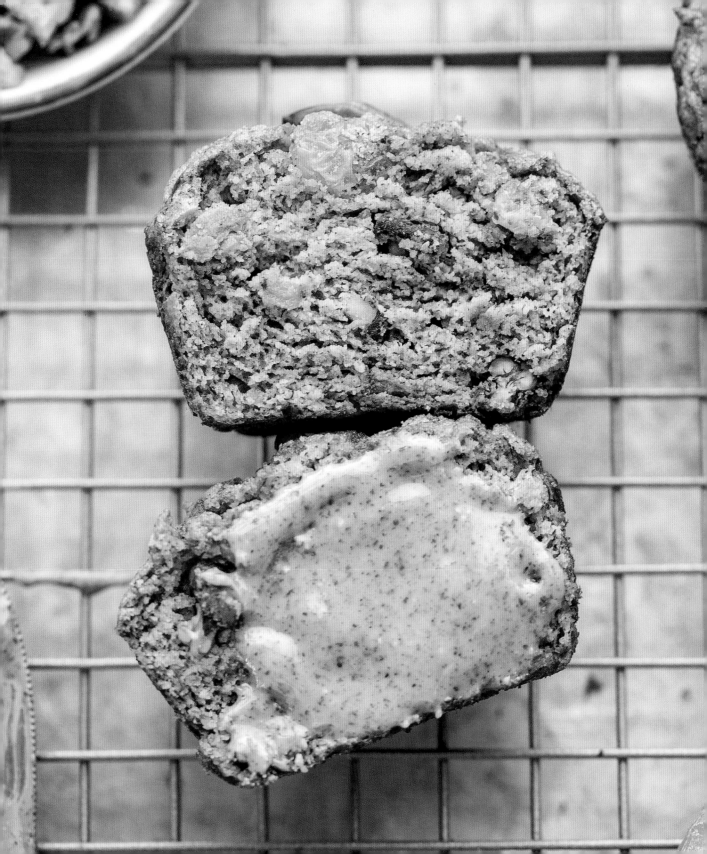

Prep time: 25 minutes

Bake time: 30 minutes

Total time: 55 minutes (plus soaking the cashews)

Yield: about 12 servings

....

1 cup (120g) raw cashews

FOR THE DOUGH

1 cup unsweetened almond milk, warmed slightly

6 tablespoons (75g) refined coconut oil, melted and cooled

1 tablespoon apple cider vinegar

1 teaspoon pure vanilla extract

3¼ cups (312g) blanched almond flour

1 cup (128g) arrowroot starch (see Tip)

1 tablespoon coconut sugar

4 teaspoons baking powder

½ teaspoon ground cinnamon

½ teaspoon kosher salt

¼ cup (20g) psyllium husks

FOR THE COATING

⅔ cup (96g) coconut sugar

2 tablespoons ground cinnamon

½ cup ghee or vegan butter, melted

FOR THE FROSTING

½ cup canned full-fat coconut milk

¼ cup (85g) pure maple syrup

1 tablespoon fresh lemon juice

½ teaspoon apple cider vinegar

¼ teaspoon vanilla bean powder

Pinch of salt

MONKEY BREAD

PALEO • GRAIN-FREE • VEGAN • GLUTEN-FREE • DAIRY-FREE

Sticky, pull-apart monkey bread was a staple of my childhood, but since going gluten-free it's been out of my diet. Traditionally, monkey bread is made with yeast dough or sometimes canned biscuits. For my version, a quick non-yeasted dough with almond flour and arrowroot starch creates soft and chewy dough balls that are then dipped in melted ghee or vegan butter and rolled in a mixture of cinnamon and coconut sugar. Baked until crispy on the top and served with a cashew-based tangy "cream cheese"–style glaze, this Monkey Bread is perfect for serving to a hungry brunch crowd. It's best when warm, and easily reheats in the oven or microwave.

....

BEFORE you begin, soak the cashews for the frosting. Put the cashews in a large bowl and add enough water to cover by 1 or 2 inches. I prefer to use filtered water but tap water is also fine. Let the cashews soak for at least 4 hours on the countertop. If soaking them longer, refrigerate for up to 12 hours. If you don't have time for the longer soak, cover the cashews with boiling water and let them soak for 1 hour. This speeds up the process although the nuts won't be as creamy as they are after a longer soak. Drain and rinse the cashews before using.

PREHEAT the oven to 375°F; grease a 9- or 8-inch Bundt pan or 8 × 8-inch baking dish (or similarly sized dish) with coconut oil.

FOR THE DOUGH: In a mixing bowl, whisk together the almond milk, coconut oil, vinegar, and vanilla to combine.

IN a separate mixing bowl, whisk together the almond flour, arrowroot starch, coconut sugar, baking powder, cinnamon, and salt.

ADD the psyllium husks to the liquid (you don't want to do this before this point or the liquid will become too thick), whisk it in, and immediately add the mixture to the dry ingredients. Use a spatula or wooden spoon to stir the mixture until a loose dough forms. It will be relatively soft and fluffy, but still easy to work with.

It shouldn't be overly sticky. If it is, add an extra tablespoon or two of arrowroot starch.

FOR THE COATING: In a small bowl, stir together the coconut sugar and cinnamon until fully combined. Put the melted vegan butter in a separate small bowl.

PLUCK about 2 teaspoons dough and roll it into a ball. Roll it in the melted butter and then in the cinnamon sugar. Continue rolling balls and coating them, arranging them in the pan and piling the balls on top of each other until all the dough is used.

BAKE for 30 to 40 minutes, until a toothpick inserted in the center of the balls comes out clean and the top is crispy. Start to check the bread for doneness at 30 minutes.

LET the monkey bread cool for about 20 minutes and then flip it out onto a plate.

FOR THE FROSTING: Drain and rinse the cashews. Combine the cashews and remaining frosting ingredients in a high-powered blender or bowl of a food processor fitted with the metal blade. Blend on medium speed for 2 to 4 minutes, until the frosting is supersmooth and creamy. Store the frosting in a tightly lidded jar in the refrigerator.

DRIZZLE the frosting over the warm monkey bread or use it as a dipping sauce.

THE monkey bread is best served warm and on the day it's made. Store leftovers in an airtight container at room temperature for up to 2 days. To reheat, warm in the oven for about 10 minutes or microwave for 30 seconds to 1 minute.

Tip

Tapioca flour can also be used, but arrowroot starch creates a better texture.

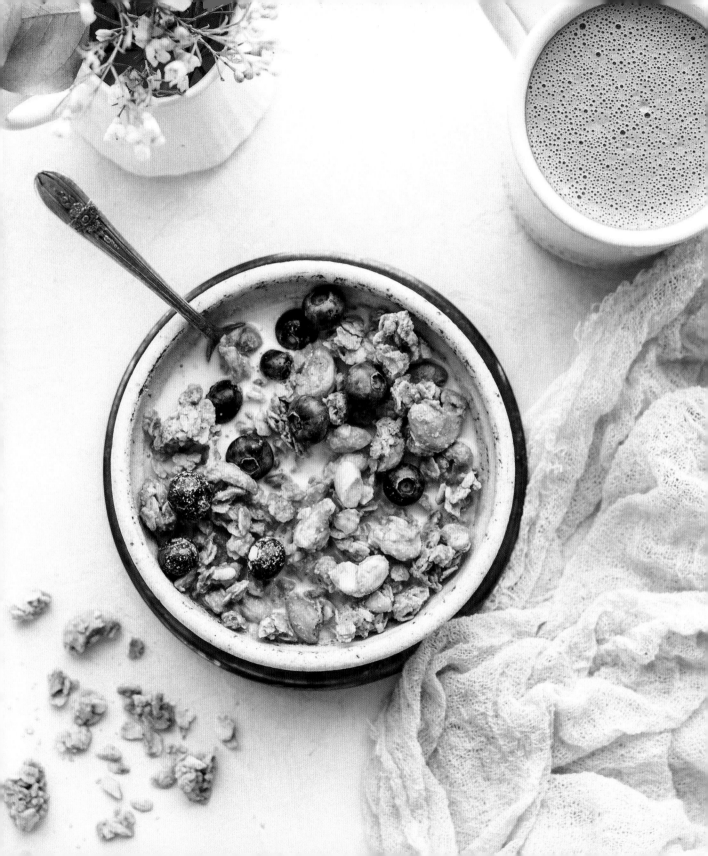

CASHEW COOKIE GRANOLA

VEGAN • GLUTEN-FREE • DAIRY-FREE

This cashew cookie granola is one of my most favorite granolas I have ever made, and I have made a lot of granola because it's one of my go-to snacks. I rarely make the same granola twice since there's so many options to experiment with. But this one—it tastes, unsurprisingly, just like a cashew cookie—is sweet but not overly so, with a warm vanilla flavor, a hint of salt, and a tender, crunchy texture. It's simple, not adorned with all kinds of nuts and seeds and dried fruit and chocolate, because it doesn't need it. The simple flavors shine. However, if you want to sass it up a bit, toss in some dried blueberries, freeze-dried strawberries or raspberries, or even chocolate chips after the granola is cooled.

Prep time: 10 minutes
Bake time: 50 minutes
Total time: 1 hour
Yield: about 5 cups

2 cups (192g) gluten-free rolled oats

1 cup (120g) roughly chopped raw cashews

½ cup (128g) cashew butter

¼ cup (85g) pure maple syrup

¼ cup (50g) refined coconut oil, melted

½ teaspoon pure vanilla extract

¼ teaspoon vanilla bean powder

½ teaspoon kosher salt

PREHEAT the oven to 300°F. Line a large (about 16 × 12-inch) baking sheet with parchment paper. Use two baking sheets if your sheets are small.

IN a large bowl, stir together the oats and cashews. In a separate, smaller mixing bowl or 2-cup liquid measuring cup, stir together the cashew butter, maple syrup, coconut oil, vanilla, vanilla bean powder, and salt until fully combined. Pour the wet ingredients over the dry ingredients and stir until the dry ingredients are completely coated.

SCRAPE the granola onto the prepared pan(s) and spread into an even layer, pressing down with your hands or a spatula. Make the granola as flat and even as you can. Bake until the granola is lightly browned, about 50 minutes, rotating the baking sheet(s) halfway through the baking time to ensure even cooking.

LET the granola cool completely on the baking sheet. Do not disturb it while cooling or you won't be able to get large pieces. When it's fully cooled, break the granola into sizable clusters. Store at room temperature in an airtight container for up to 1 month, if it lasts that long!

Prep time: 10 minutes
Chill time: 1 hour
Total time: 1 hour 10 minutes
Yield: 10 bars

1½ cups (144g) gluten-free quick-cooking oats

1½ cups (42g) crispy brown rice cereal

½ cup (56g) sliced almonds, toasted

⅓ cup (67g) refined coconut oil

⅓ cup (113g) pure maple syrup

⅓ cup (85g) creamy almond butter

½ teaspoon pure vanilla extract

¼ teaspoon kosher salt

½ cup freeze-dried raspberries, lightly crushed

2 ounces (57g) bittersweet chocolate (optional but recommended)

RASPBERRY–ALMOND BUTTER GRANOLA BARS

VEGAN • NO-BAKE • GLUTEN-FREE • DAIRY-FREE

Remember chewy granola bars, the staple of lunch boxes everywhere? These raspberry bars remind me so much of them—the light, chewy texture, the almond butter mixture that holds it all together, and the drizzle of chocolate on top. These have a flavor upgrade, though—while the classic chocolate chip is good, I think almond butter and freeze-dried raspberries make them so much better. The crunchy berries add a hint of tartness that plays perfectly with the richness of the almond butter and the drizzle of chocolate. These, too, are perfect for lunch boxes everywhere, but you'll feel better knowing exactly what went into them!

LINE an 8 × 8-inch baking pan with parchment paper.

IN a large bowl, stir the oats with the cereal and almonds.

IN a small saucepan, heat the coconut oil and maple syrup over medium-low heat until just starting to boil, stirring frequently. Boil for 1 minute longer, then remove the pan from the heat. Add the almond butter, vanilla, and salt and stir until smooth.

POUR the hot mixture over the oat mixture and mix until thoroughly combined. Stir in the freeze-dried raspberries.

SCRAPE the granola mixture into the pan and spread evenly. Refrigerate for about 1 hour. When set, use a sharp knife to cut into 10 bars.

IF using the chocolate, chop it into large pieces and transfer to a microwave-safe container. Microwave for about 30 seconds. Stir until the chocolate is liquid and smooth. Microwave for another 30 seconds, if needed. Spoon the melted chocolate into a piping bag, or into a zippered plastic bag and then snip off a corner. Drizzle over the bars. Refrigerate for about 15 minutes, until set.

TO store, tightly wrap the bars in plastic wrap or place in an airtight container and refrigerate for up to 2 weeks (best within the first 4 days, though).

LEMON-BLUEBERRY BREAKFAST CAKE

PALEO • GRAIN-FREE • VEGAN • GLUTEN-FREE • DAIRY-FREE

A little chewy, a little cakey, and fully delicious, this simple breakfast cake is as easy to make as it is to eat. The bright summery flavors of lemon and blueberry make the cake incredibly flavorful with a unique texture that will keep you coming back for more. I love serving this with coffee or tea for brunch, but it also makes a scrumptious dessert. Don't forget the lemony glaze on top—it contributes a beautiful brightness. If fresh blueberries aren't in season, frozen can be used. Just make sure to thaw and drain them before using to avoid adding too much moisture.

FOR THE CAKE: Preheat the oven to 350°F. Line an 8 × 8-inch baking pan with parchment paper and grease with coconut oil.

IN a bowl, stir together the cashew butter, coconut oil, coconut sugar, flax egg, lemon zest and juice, and vanilla until smooth and combined. Stir in the coconut flour, baking soda, and salt. Fold in the blueberries.

SPREAD the batter evenly in the prepared pan. Bake for 22 to 24 minutes, until a toothpick inserted in the center comes out clean. Cool completely in the pan set on a wire rack.

FOR THE GLAZE: Combine the coconut butter, coconut oil, and maple syrup in a microwave-safe bowl and microwave for 30 seconds. Stir the mixture, making sure the butter melts. If necessary, microwave for another 30 seconds and stir again. The mixture might seize up, but don't worry, the lemon juice will thin it out! (The mixture can also be heated in a small saucepan over low heat.) Slowly whisk the lemon juice into the glaze until it's thinned to your liking.

REMOVE the cake from the pan, set on the wire rack or a plate, and spread the glaze over the cake. Refrigerate for about 1 hour to give the glaze time to firm up, then cut with a sharp knife.

STORE the cake in an airtight container in the refrigerator for up to 1 week, or in the freezer for up to 3 months.

Prep time: 15 minutes
Bake time: 22 minutes
Chill time: 1 hour
Total time: 1 hour 37 minutes
Yield: 8 to 10 servings

FOR THE CAKE
½ cup (128g) cashew or almond butter

¼ cup (50g) refined coconut oil, melted

¾ cup (108g) coconut sugar

1 flax egg (see Tip) or 1 large egg

Grated zest of 1 lemon

2 tablespoons fresh lemon juice

1 teaspoon pure vanilla extract

½ cup (64g) coconut flour

½ teaspoon baking soda

¼ teaspoon kosher salt

⅔ cup fresh blueberries (about ½ pint)

FOR THE GLAZE
¼ cup (64g) coconut butter

1 tablespoon refined coconut oil

1 tablespoon pure maple syrup or honey

¼ cup fresh lemon juice

Tip

To make the flax egg, whisk 2 tablespoons ground flax seed with 2½ tablespoons water. Let stand for 10 minutes to gel.

Prep time: 15 minutes
Cook time: 2 minutes
Chill time: 1 hour
Total time: 1 hour 17 minutes
Yield: 10 granola bars

- 1¼ cups (178g) finely chopped unsalted roasted peanuts
- 1¼ cups (75g) finely chopped flaked coconut
- ⅔ cup (172g) creamy peanut butter
- ¼ cup (84g) pure maple syrup
- 2 tablespoons virgin coconut oil
- 2 tablespoons Toasted Coconut Butter (page 265)
- 1 teaspoon pure vanilla extract
- ½ teaspoon kosher salt

FOR THE OPTIONAL GLAZE
- 2 tablespoons Toasted Coconut Butter (page 265)
- 1 tablespoon creamy peanut butter

COCONUT–PEANUT BUTTER GRAIN-FREE GRANOLA BARS

GRAIN-FREE • VEGAN • NO-BAKE • GLUTEN-FREE • DAIRY-FREE

These grain-free bars are loaded with healthy fats to keep you fueled all day long thanks to the peanuts, peanut butter, coconut, coconut oil, and coconut butter. Finely chopped peanuts and flaked coconut are the perfect grain-free replacement for oats, which are typically the base of granola bars. The bars can also easily be made Paleo-friendly by replacing the peanuts and peanut butter with your favorite Paleo nut—almonds and almond butter would be great.

LINE an 8 × 8-inch baking pan with parchment paper and grease lightly with coconut oil.

IN a large mixing bowl, stir the peanuts and flaked coconut together.

IN a small saucepan, combine the peanut butter, maple syrup, and coconut oil and bring to a boil over medium heat. Let the mixture simmer rapidly and bubble for 2 minutes. Remove the pan from the heat and stir in the coconut butter, vanilla, and salt, whisking until the coconut butter melts into the mixture (if it wasn't already melty).

POUR the peanut butter–maple syrup mixture over the dry ingredients and stir until the dry ingredients are well coated.

POUR and scrape this sticky mixture into the prepared pan. Use a rubber spatula to press the mixture into a firm, even layer that covers the bottom of the pan. Cover with plastic wrap and refrigerate for at least 1 hour, then use a sharp knife to cut into 10 granola bars.

GLAZE the granola bars. If you are glazing the bars, microwave the toasted coconut butter in a small microwave-safe bowl for 30 seconds, then stir until smooth. Whisk in the peanut butter. Transfer the mixture to a piping bag or small zippered plastic bag with a corner snipped. Drizzle over the bars. Return the bars to the refrigerator for about 10 minutes to firm up.

WRAP the bars individually, or put them in an airtight container and refrigerate for up to 2 weeks or freeze for up to 3 months. Do not leave the bars at room temperature for more than 1 hour or they will soften.

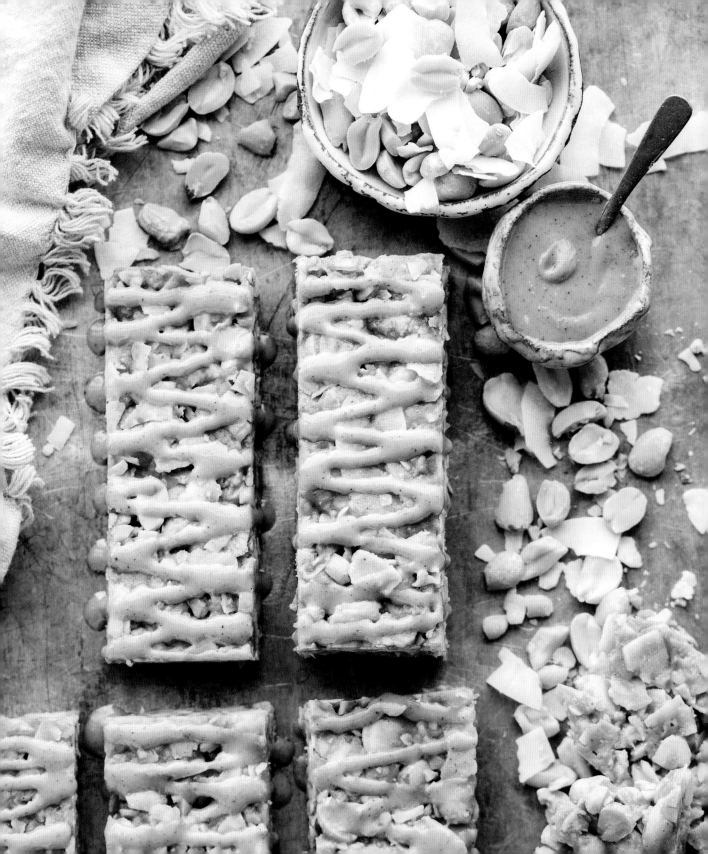

Prep time: 20 minutes

Chill time: 1 hour

Bake time: 30 minutes

Total time: 1 hour 50 minutes

Yield: 18 mini scones or 8 larger scones

FOR THE EVERYTHING BAGEL SEASONING

1 tablespoon poppy seeds

1 tablespoon white sesame seeds

1 tablespoon black sesame seeds

1 tablespoon dried minced garlic

1 tablespoon dried minced onion

2 teaspoons coarse salt

FOR THE SCONES

2¼ cups (216g) blanched almond flour

¾ cup (96g) arrowroot starch, plus more for dusting

1 tablespoon nutritional yeast

1¼ teaspoons baking powder

½ teaspoon sea salt

½ cup (100g) refined coconut oil, solid

½ cup canned full-fat coconut milk, plus extra to brush on top of the scones

1 flax egg (see Tip)

Tip

To make the flax egg, whisk 2 tablespoons ground flax seed with 2½ tablespoons water. Let stand for 10 minutes to gel.

EVERYTHING BAGEL SCONES

PALEO • GRAIN-FREE • VEGAN • GLUTEN-FREE • DAIRY-FREE

Since Trader Joe's came out with Everything But the Bagel Seasoning, I've been seeing everything bagel–flavored everything. I'm not mad about it—it's a beyond delicious flavor combination. I'm throwing my hat into the ring with these everything bagel scones, which are deliciously savory from the seasoning and nutritional yeast (which adds a cheesy, umami flavor), and have a texture that is tender and flaky with crispy edges. The mini scones are so good slathered with a little bit of vegan butter, ghee, or dairy-free cream cheese, or make larger scones and use them like toast! If you don't feel like making the everything bagel seasoning, buy it at the supermarket.

FOR THE EVERYTHING BAGEL SEASONING: Stir together all ingredients. Store in a small, lidded jar. Makes 6 tablespoons, which is more than you need for this recipe but the seasoning keeps and you can use it for other things.

FOR THE SCONES: In the bowl of a food processor fitted with the metal blade or a large mixing bowl, pulse or whisk 2 tablespoons seasoning, the almond flour, arrowroot starch, nutritional yeast, baking powder, and salt. Add the coconut oil and pulse or use a pastry cutter or fork to work the coconut oil into the dry ingredients until only small bits of coconut oil remain.

IN a small mixing bowl, whisk together the coconut milk and flax egg. Add to the dry ingredients and pulse or stir until completely combined.

PUT a sheet of parchment paper on a baking sheet and dust with arrowroot starch. Put the dough on the parchment, dust with more arrowroot starch, and press into a 7- or 8-inch square, about ¾ inch thick. If you'd rather make 8 larger scones, form the dough into an 8-inch round about 1 inch thick. Refrigerate until chilled, about 1 hour.

WHEN ready to bake, preheat the oven to 375°F. Cut the square into nine 2½-inch squares, then cut each diagonally to make 18 scones. If you're making larger scones, cut the rounds into quarters and then cut each in half to make 8 triangles. Separate the scones from each other on the baking sheet just so they're not touching.

BRUSH each scone with coconut milk and then sprinkle with more everything bagel seasoning. Bake until the scones are golden brown, 20 to 30 minutes, depending on the size of the scones.

SERVE the scones warm. Refrigerate in an airtight container for up to 1 week.

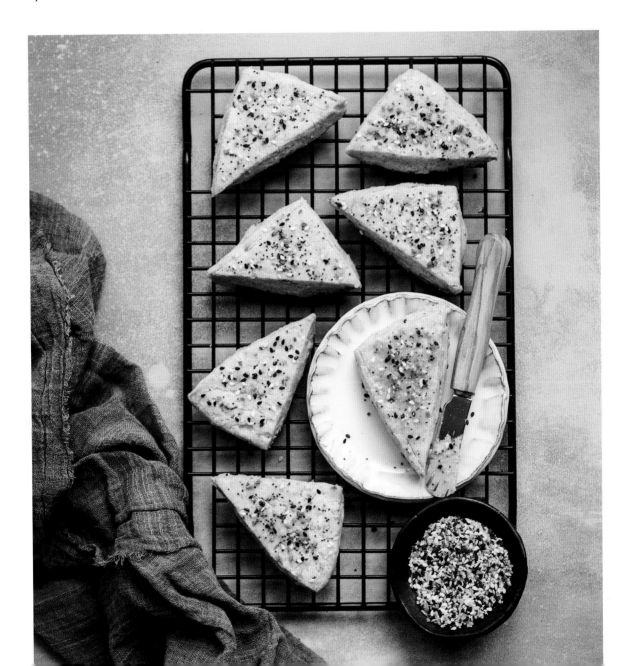

CHAPTER TWO

Cakes, Cupcakes, and Cheesecakes

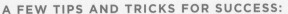

A FEW TIPS AND TRICKS FOR SUCCESS:

For the baked cakes and cupcakes in this chapter, make sure all of your ingredients are at room temperature or slightly warm, including the eggs and milk, otherwise the melted coconut oil will harden up and mess up the batter.

Baking times can vary for a variety of reasons, many times due to inaccurate oven temperatures, so make sure a toothpick comes out clean and the cake (or cupcake or loaf) springs back when pressed with a finger. If you press and an indent stays, let the cake bake for a few more minutes. Even better, get an oven thermometer to ensure you're baking at the correct temperature.

Many recipes in this chapter (such as the cheesecakes and the frostings) call for soaked cashews, so make sure you begin to soak them at least 4 hours ahead of time. If you don't have 4 hours, you can cover the cashews with boiling water for 1 hour to speed up this process.

When baking cakes and cupcakes, be sure to leave the oven door closed throughout the baking process. Opening the door too early can release too much heat and cause the cake or cupcakes to sink in the center.

Prep time: 30 minutes

Bake time: 18 minutes

Total time: 48 minutes (plus soaking the cashews)

Yield: 12 cupcakes

....

1½ cups (180g) raw cashews

FOR THE CUPCAKES

1 cup plus 2 tablespoons (108g) blanched almond flour

⅓ cup (38g) tapioca flour

½ teaspoon baking soda

½ teaspoon baking powder

¾ teaspoon kosher salt

¾ cup (108g) coconut sugar

½ cup (42g) unsweetened cocoa powder

¼ cup (61g) unsweetened applesauce

⅓ cup dairy-free milk, such as unsweetened almond milk

2 large eggs, at room temperature

¼ cup (50g) refined coconut oil, melted

1 teaspoon pure vanilla extract

FOR THE SALTED CASHEW FROSTING

⅓ cup canned full-fat coconut milk

¼ cup refined coconut oil, melted

¼ cup pure maple syrup

¼ cup creamy roasted cashew butter (see Tip)

½ teaspoon pure vanilla extract

¼ teaspoon sea salt

CONTINUES

CHOCOLATE CUPCAKES WITH SALTED CASHEW FROSTING

PALEO • GRAIN-FREE • GLUTEN-FREE • DAIRY-FREE

I couldn't write a cookbook without including the classics, and it doesn't get much more classic than chocolate cupcakes. These are light, fluffy, and full of chocolate flavor. They're perfectly complemented by the creamy salted cashew frosting, which is made with soaked cashews and roasted cashew butter. I like drizzling No-Cook Caramel Sauce on top of the frosting and adding a sprinkle of sea salt to make the cupcakes extra decadent. Or simply top with sprinkles and these are perfect for a birthday party!

....

BEFORE you begin, soak the cashews for the frosting. Put the cashews in a large bowl and add enough water to cover by 1 or 2 inches. I prefer to use filtered water but tap water is also fine. Let the cashews soak for at least 4 hours on the countertop. If soaking for longer, refrigerate for up to 12 hours. If you don't have time for the longer soak, cover the cashews with boiling water and let them soak for 1 hour. This speeds up the process although the nuts won't be as creamy as after a longer soak. Drain and rinse the cashews before using.

FOR THE CUPCAKES: Preheat the oven to 350°F; line one 12-cup muffin tin or two 6-cup muffin tins with paper liners.

IN a large mixing bowl, whisk together the almond flour, tapioca flour, baking soda, baking powder, salt, coconut sugar, and cocoa powder.

IN a separate mixing bowl, whisk together the applesauce, almond milk, eggs, coconut oil, and vanilla extract until smooth.

POUR the wet ingredients into the dry ingredients and stir until well combined.

SPOON the batter into the cupcake liners, filling each about two-thirds full. Bake for about 18 minutes, until a toothpick inserted into the center of a cupcake comes out clean and the tops of the

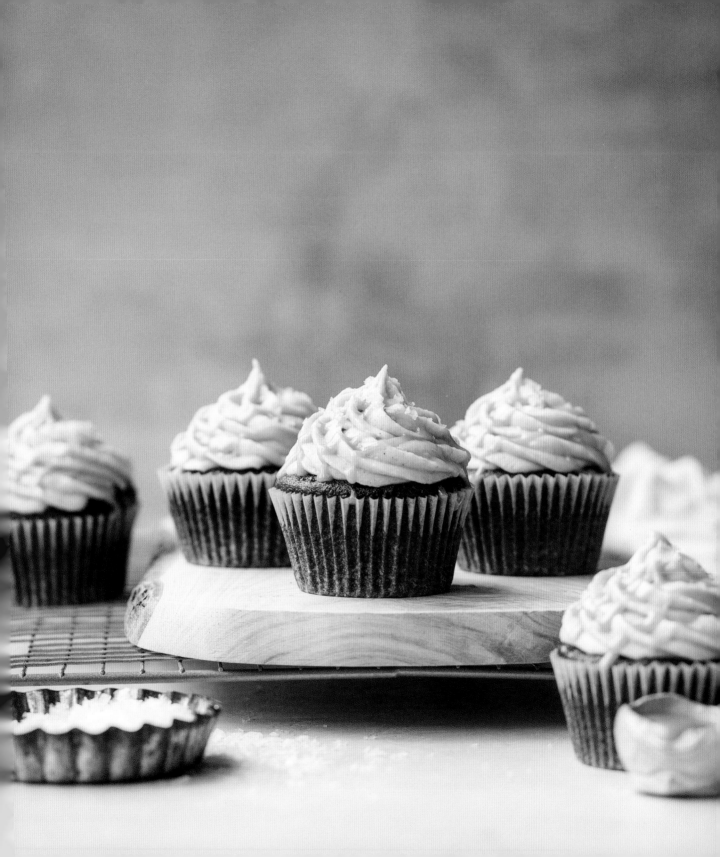

TO GARNISH
No-Cook Caramel Sauce
   (page 277)

Flaky sea salt

Tip

The cashew butter in the frosting can be replaced with any nut butter you prefer. Peanut butter would be delicious!

cupcakes spring back when gently pressed with your fingertip. Set the cupcake tin on a wire rack to cool completely before removing the cupcakes from the tin.

FOR THE FROSTING: Drain and rinse the cashews. In a high-powered blender such as a Vitamix, or a bowl of a food processor fitted with a metal blade, blend the drained cashews and the remaining frosting ingredients until smooth and creamy, 3 to 5 minutes. Use the tamper for the blender or scrape down the sides of the bowl as needed to ensure the frosting blends smoothly.

IF you want a thin spread of frosting, frost the cupcakes with the frosting as it is at this point.

IF you'd like to pipe the frosting, transfer it to a metal bowl and refrigerate for at least 1 hour, until it's thick enough to pipe on top of the cupcakes. If you'd like the frosting to be a little fluffier, transfer to a stand mixer fitted with the whisk attachment (or use a hand mixer) and mix it for about 30 seconds. Transfer the thickened or fluffy frosting to a piping bag fitted with a star tip or a zippered plastic bag with the corner snipped off and pipe the frosting on the cupcakes.

AFTER frosting the cupcakes, garnish with a drizzle of caramel sauce and a sprinkle of flaky sea salt, if desired.

STORE the cupcakes in an airtight container in the refrigerator for up to 5 days.

SHAINA'S BIRTHDAY CAKE

PALEO • GRAIN-FREE • GLUTEN-FREE • DAIRY-FREE

Before my sister's 28th birthday, she called me to request a birthday cake. Being gluten-free and refined sugar–free, she hadn't had a birthday cake in many years. She requested a healthier Funfetti cake, with cream and strawberries—a favorite from childhood, just made more wholesome. I whipped up the cake and brought it to the restaurant where we were celebrating . . . and as soon as I walked in the door, the staff was not happy about having a homemade cake on the premises. They took it back to the refrigerator and told us we were not allowed to eat the cake there, despite them not having any desserts on the menu that my sister could eat. At the end of the meal, they brought the cake back for us to take home, and that's when my dad produced a handful of forks he had stashed in his pocket. We tore into the sides of the cake, no slicing or plates, much to the dismay of our side-eyeing waitress. The illicit nature of our cake eating made it even more enjoyable. I re-created the cake here, and it's one of my favorites in the book: a soft and sweet vanilla-scented cake, with layers of fluffy coconut cream and fresh strawberries. It's light, beautiful, and perfect for summer.

PREHEAT the oven to 350°F. Line two 8-inch round cake pans or three 6-inch round cake pans with parchment paper and grease with coconut oil.

FOR THE CAKE: In a large mixing bowl, whisk the almond flour with the tapioca flour, baking soda, baking powder, salt, coconut sugar, and vanilla bean powder. (If using extract, add it to the liquid ingredients.)

IN a separate mixing bowl, whisk together the applesauce, vinegar, milk, melted coconut oil, and eggs (and extract if using). Pour the wet ingredients into the dry ingredients and stir until well combined.

DIVIDE the batter evenly among the pans. Bake for 25 to 30 minutes, depending on the pan size, until a toothpick inserted near the center of the layers comes out clean and the cake springs back when gently pressed. Start checking the three 6-inch

CONTINUES

Prep time: 45 minutes
Bake time: 30 minutes
Total time: 1¼ hours
Yield: about 10 slices

FOR THE CAKE

3 cups (288g) blanched almond flour

⅔ cup (76g) tapioca flour

1 teaspoon baking soda

1 teaspoon baking powder

1 teaspoon kosher salt

1⅓ cups (192g) coconut sugar

¾ teaspoon vanilla bean powder, or 2 teaspoons pure vanilla extract

⅔ cup (162g) unsweetened applesauce

1 teaspoon apple cider vinegar

½ cup dairy-free milk, such as unsweetened almond milk, warmed slightly

6 tablespoons (75g) refined coconut oil, melted and cooled

4 large eggs, at room temperature

FOR THE FILLING

3 (13.5-ounce) cans full-fat coconut cream, chilled overnight

2 tablespoons pure maple syrup

¼ teaspoon vanilla bean powder, or 1 teaspoon vanilla extract

About 2 cups sliced fresh strawberries (from about 1 pint; amount will depend on number of cake layers)

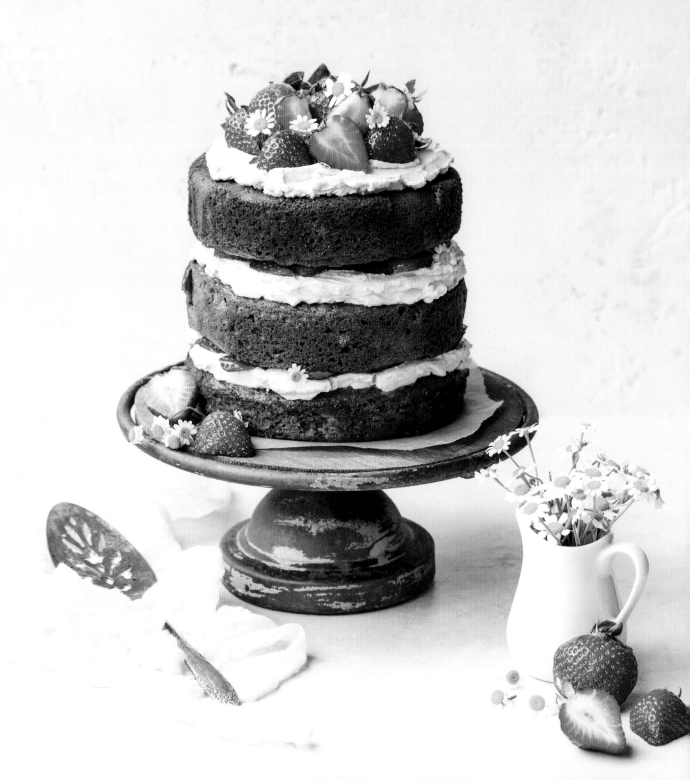

layers after 20 or 21 minutes and the two 8-inch layers after 25 or 26 minutes. Let the layers cool completely in the pans set on wire racks before removing them.

FOR THE FILLING: Drain any liquid from the cans of coconut cream and transfer the thick cream to a mixing bowl or the bowl of a stand mixer. Whip until smooth and fluffy, then add the maple syrup and vanilla bean powder. Mix until combined.

TO ASSEMBLE THE CAKE: If any of the layers dome, trim the tops to make them level. Divide the filling and strawberries into two or three portions, depending on the number of cake layers. Place one cooled cake layer, trimmed side up, on a cake stand (or whatever you'd like to serve it on). Top the layer with one portion of the filling and then cover with one portion of the fresh strawberry slices.

TOP with the second cake layer and repeat with the filling and strawberries. If you have a third layer, position it on top and spread the rest of the filling (now frosting) over it and top with the remaining sliced strawberries.

SERVE at once or cover and refrigerate for up to 5 days.

If you want to make the cake Funfetti style, stir about ¼ cup of naturally colored sprinkles into the batter!

Prep time: 30 minutes

Chill time: 4 hours

Total time: 4½ hours (plus soaking the cashews)

Yield: 10 slices

---

2 cups (240g) raw cashews

FOR THE CRUST

½ cup (60g) raw cashews

½ cup (48g) blanched almond flour

2 Medjool dates, pitted

2 tablespoons (25g) refined coconut oil

¼ teaspoon kosher salt

FOR THE CHEESECAKE FILLING

½ cup shaken canned full-fat coconut milk

⅓ cup pure maple syrup

3 tablespoons cacao butter, melted

1 tablespoon fresh lemon juice

1 tablespoon vanilla extract, or ½ teaspoon vanilla bean powder

½ teaspoon apple cider vinegar

½ cup freeze-dried raspberries

FOR THE RASPBERRY LAYER

1 cup fresh or frozen raspberries (see Tip)

1 tablespoon fresh lemon juice

2 teaspoons chia seeds

WHITE CHOCOLATE–RASPBERRY CHEESECAKE

PALEO • GRAIN-FREE • VEGAN • NO-BAKE • GLUTEN-FREE • DAIRY-FREE

When I first went dairy-free, I mourned the loss of white chocolate. I had never seen or heard of dairy-free white chocolate—it seemed to be impossible to make without milk. Then I discovered that the flavor of white chocolate could be created with some cacao butter and vanilla! This white chocolate–raspberry cheesecake was born out of my cacao butter experiments and is one of my favorites. It is lusciously rich from the cacao butter and has a sweet, tangy flavor thanks to the raspberries. You can make it even more irresistible by opting for vanilla bean powder in place of vanilla extract, which adds beautiful vanilla bean flecks to the mix.

BEFORE you begin, soak the cashews for the filling. Put the cashews in a large bowl and add enough water to cover by 1 or 2 inches. I prefer to use filtered water but tap water is also fine. Let the cashews soak for at least 4 hours on the countertop. If soaking them longer, refrigerate for up to 12 hours. If you don't have time for the longer soak, cover the cashews with boiling water and let them soak for 1 hour. This speeds up the process, although the nuts won't be as creamy as after a longer soak. Drain and rinse the cashews before using.

FOR THE CRUST: Grease a 6-inch springform pan or an 8-inch square baking pan with coconut oil and place a round of parchment paper in the bottom for easy removal. Alternatively, you can line a 6-inch cake pan with strips of parchment paper laid across the pan, creating a sort of sling to help with removal. Lightly grease the parchment and pan with coconut oil.

COMBINE the ½ cup cashews, almond flour, dates, coconut oil, and salt in the bowl of a food processor fitted with the metal blade or a high-powered blender (I use a Vitamix). Pulse until the ingredients come together as a sticky dough. Don't overprocess or it will turn into nut butter! Press the dough into a flat crust on the bottom of the prepared pan.

CONTINUES

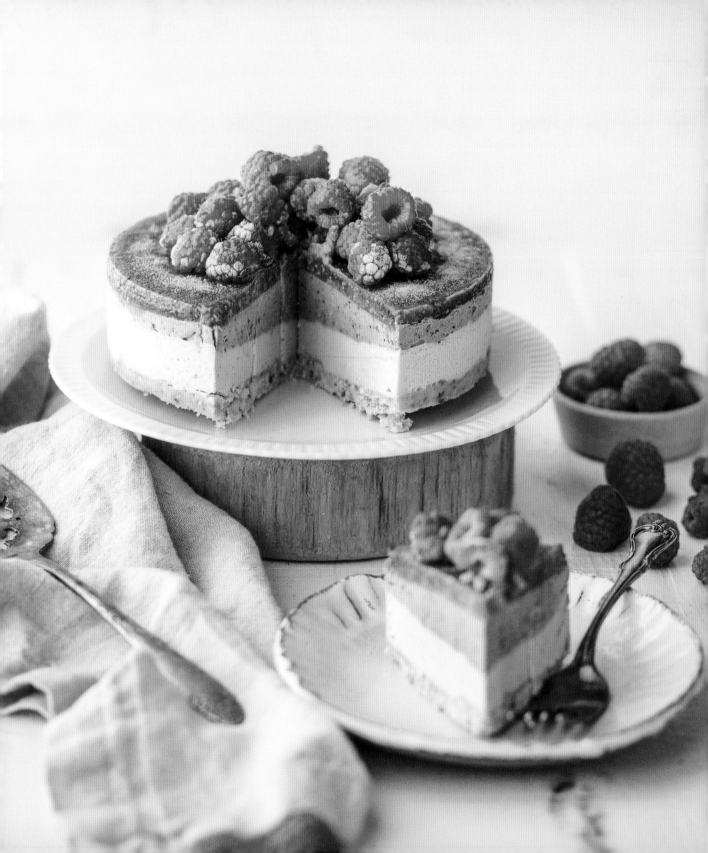

Tip

FOR THE CHEESECAKE FILLING: Drain and rinse the soaked cashews. In the same food processor or high-powered blender (no need to wash between), combine the drained cashews with the coconut milk, maple syrup, cacao butter, lemon juice, vanilla, and vinegar. Blend for 2 to 3 minutes, until the mixture is a silky smooth and super-creamy batter. Scrape down the sides of the food processor or blender canister as necessary.

POUR two-thirds of the filling over the crust; reserve the remaining filling. Smooth out the top and tap the pan hard against the counter a few times to release any air bubbles. Put the cheesecake in the freezer to firm up while finishing the rest of the cheesecake.

ADD the freeze-dried raspberries to the reserved filling and blend to incorporate. Spread this mixture over the vanilla layer and return it to the freezer.

FOR THE RASPBERRY LAYER: Rinse out the food processor or blender and add the fresh or frozen raspberries, lemon juice, and chia seeds. Blend until the raspberries are pureed. Pour them over the other layers in the pan. Freeze until completely firm, about 4 hours.

WHEN you're ready to serve, let the cheesecake thaw at room temperature for 10 to 15 minutes before slicing. I recommend running your knife under hot water to warm it up and drying it before cutting the cake with the still-hot knife. Store tightly wrapped in the freezer for up to 2 months. You can also keep the cheesecake in the fridge for up to 5 days.

VANILLA BEAN CUPCAKES WITH BANANA FROSTING

PALEO • GRAIN-FREE • GLUTEN-FREE • DAIRY-FREE

These vanilla bean cupcakes are my favorite vanilla cupcakes of all time. Because even though they're "vanilla," they certainly aren't boring. I use vanilla bean powder for maximum vanilla flavor, which also means there are tiny vanilla bean flecks throughout the cake. Since the cupcakes are sweetened with coconut sugar they aren't as pale as the vanilla cupcakes you're used to, but the coconut sugar adds a decadent caramel flavor that makes them even more irresistible. I top them with a banana-flavored cashew frosting, but since it's made with freeze-dried bananas, you can substitute any freeze-dried berry of your choice to make them your own!

BEFORE you begin, soak the cashews for the frosting. Put the cashews in a large bowl and add enough water to cover by 1 or 2 inches. I prefer to use filtered water but tap water is also fine. Let the cashews soak for at least 4 hours on the countertop. If soaking longer, refrigerate for up to 12 hours. If you don't have time for the longer soak, cover the cashews with boiling water and let them soak for 1 hour. This speeds up the process although the nuts won't be as creamy as after a longer soak. Drain and rinse the cashews before using.

PREHEAT the oven to 350°F; line 11 cups of a 12-cup muffin pan with paper liners.

FOR THE CUPCAKES: In a large mixing bowl, whisk the almond flour with the tapioca flour, baking soda, baking powder, salt, coconut sugar, and vanilla bean powder. (If using extract, add it to the liquid ingredients.)

IN a separate mixing bowl, stir together the mashed banana, vinegar, milk, eggs, melted coconut oil, and vanilla extract if using. Pour the wet ingredients into the dry ingredients and stir until combined.

USE a spoon or large cookie scoop to fill the cupcake cups, filling each about two-thirds full. Bake for 16 to 18 minutes, until a

Prep time: 10 minutes
Bake time: 16 minutes
Total time: 26 minutes (plus soaking the cashews)
Yield: 11 cupcakes

1½ cups (180g) raw cashews

FOR THE CUPCAKES
1½ cups (144g) blanched almond flour
⅓ cup (38g) tapioca flour
½ teaspoon baking soda
½ teaspoon baking powder
½ teaspoon kosher salt
⅔ cup (96g) coconut sugar
¾ teaspoon vanilla bean powder, or 2 teaspoons vanilla extract
⅓ cup mashed ripe banana (see Tip)
½ teaspoon apple cider vinegar
¼ cup dairy-free milk, such as unsweetened almond milk, warmed slightly
2 large eggs, at room temperature
3 tablespoons (38g) refined coconut oil, melted and cooled

FOR THE FROSTING
¼ cup canned coconut cream
¼ cup refined coconut oil, melted
¼ cup pure maple syrup
1 tablespoon fresh lemon juice
½ teaspoon vanilla extract
½ cup freeze-dried bananas
½ teaspoon ground cinnamon
Pinch of salt (optional)

CONTINUES

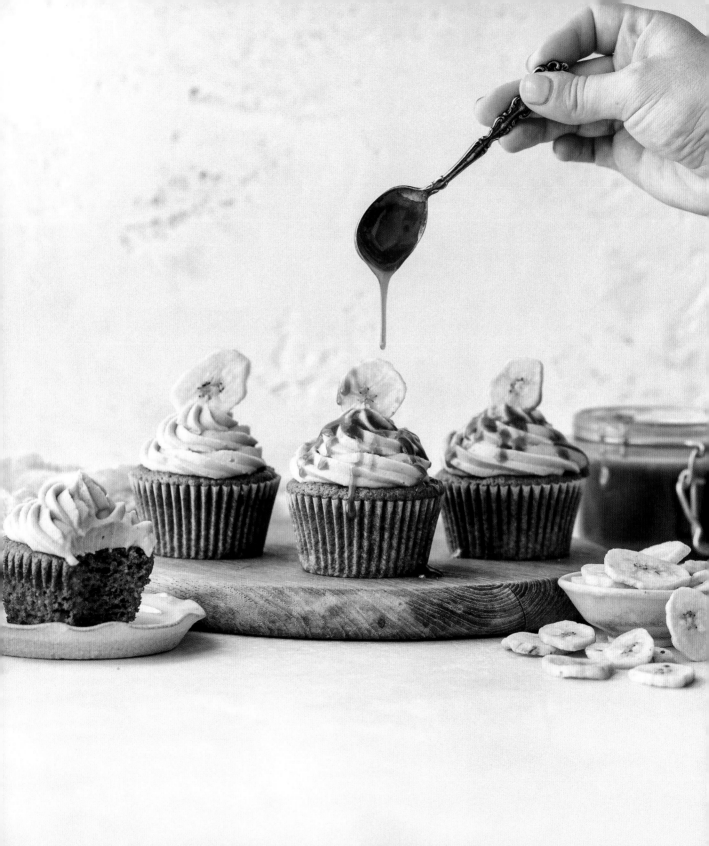

toothpick inserted in the center of a cupcake comes out clean and the tops of the cupcakes spring back when gently pressed. Set the cupcake tin on a wire rack and let the cupcakes cool completely.

FOR THE FROSTING: Meanwhile, drain the cashews and rinse with cool water. In a high-powered blender (I use a Vitamix) or the bowl of a food processor fitted with the metal blade, blend the drained cashews until they are smooth and creamy. Add the rest of the frosting ingredients except the salt and blend for 3 to 5 minutes, until as smooth and creamy as possible. Taste and add the salt, if needed.

IF you're just spreading the frosting on the cupcakes, you can frost them now. If you'd prefer to pipe the frosting on the cupcakes, transfer the frosting to a bowl and refrigerate for about 1 hour, whisking every 20 minutes, until it's thickened enough to pipe on the cupcakes. Spoon the frosting into a piping bag or plastic bag with a corner snipped off and pipe it over the cooled cupcakes.

AFTER frosting them, garnish the cupcakes with a sprinkle of cinnamon or a drizzle of caramel sauce, if desired.

REFRIGERATE the cupcakes, tightly sealed, for up to 3 days, or freeze unfrosted cupcakes for up to 2 months.

FOR OPTIONAL GARNISH
Ground cinnamon

Salted Caramel Sauce
   (page 270)

Tip

You can use applesauce in place of the banana for a more neutral flavor.

Prep time: 15 minutes
Bake time: 30 minutes
Total time: 45 minutes
Yield: 8 slices

FOR THE CAKE

2 cups (192g) blanched almond flour

⅓ cup (43g) coconut flour

¼ cup (32g) arrowroot starch

⅔ cup (96g) coconut sugar

½ cup (42g) cacao powder

1½ teaspoons baking powder

1 teaspoon baking soda

1 teaspoon instant espresso powder

1 teaspoon kosher salt

1 ounce (28g) unsweetened chocolate, chopped

1 cup unsweetened almond milk, warmed slightly

¼ cup (50g) olive oil

¼ cup (85g) pure maple syrup

2 flax eggs (see Tip)

1 teaspoon pure vanilla extract

FOR THE GANACHE

5 ounces bittersweet chocolate, chopped or in chips (about ¾ cup)

½ cup canned full-fat coconut milk

Tip

To make 2 flax eggs, whisk 2 tablespoons ground flax seed with 5 tablespoons water. Let set for 10 minutes to gel.

VEGAN CHOCOLATE CAKE WITH RICH CHOCOLATE GANACHE

PALEO • GRAIN-FREE • VEGAN • GLUTEN-FREE • DAIRY-FREE

Ah, chocolate cake. One of life's best pleasures, and forever one of my favorite things to eat on this planet. The second I started working on this book, a chocolate cake was on the list. But I wanted the chocolate cake to be both Paleo and vegan, as well as absurdly delicious. I tested this so many times, and almost gave up so many times, until I finally nailed the recipe—a moist, decadent, über-chocolatey cake, dripping with a smooth and rich chocolate ganache. My dad compared the cake to the Entenmann's cakes he loved in his childhood, but this one is certainly the more wholesome option. This cake has been raved about by everyone who has tried it, and I hope you love it as much as we did!

PREHEAT the oven to 350°F; lightly grease a small (8- to 9-inch) Bundt pan with coconut oil.

FOR THE CAKE: In a large mixing bowl, whisk the almond flour, coconut flour, arrowroot starch, coconut sugar, cacao powder, baking powder, baking soda, espresso powder, and salt.

MICROWAVE the 1 ounce chopped chocolate in a small, microwave-safe bowl for about 20 seconds, until softened. Stir the chocolate to liquefy it. In a separate bowl, stir together the melted chocolate, almond milk, olive oil, maple syrup, flax eggs, and vanilla extract.

POUR the liquid ingredients over the dry ingredients and stir well to mix thoroughly. Scrape the cake batter into the prepared pan and smooth the surface with a rubber spatula or spoon.

BAKE for 30 to 40 minutes, until a toothpick inserted in the center comes out clean and the cake springs back when pressed lightly.

LET the cake cool for about 30 minutes in the pan before turning out or releasing the cake onto a wire rack resting in a baking sheet to catch the ganache.

FOR THE GANACHE: In a microwave-safe bowl, combine the chocolate and coconut milk. Microwave for 1 minute, let the ganache sit for 1 minute, and then whisk until smooth. If it's not fully melted, microwave for another 20 seconds and stir again. Pour the ganache over the cooled cake, guiding it with a knife so that it covers the top of the cake and some drips down the sides.

THE cake will keep under a cake dome or in an airtight container at room temperature for 3 days, or in the refrigerator for 1 week.

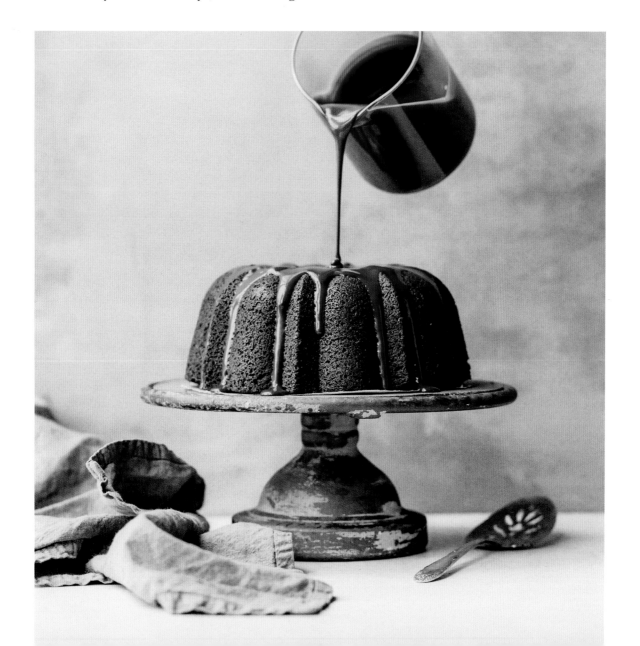

Prep time: 20 minutes

Bake time: 22 minutes

Total time: 42 minutes (plus soaking the cashews)

Yield: 16 squares

....

1 cup (120g) raw cashews

FOR THE CAKE

½ cup (128g) creamy cashew or almond butter

½ cup (72g) coconut sugar

¼ cup (50g) refined coconut oil, melted

¼ cup (61g) unsweetened applesauce

1 teaspoon pure vanilla extract

¾ cup (72g) blanched almond flour

¼ cup (32g) coconut flour

¾ teaspoon baking powder

1 teaspoon ground cinnamon

¼ teaspoon kosher salt

¾ cup freshly grated (see Tip) carrots (2 to 3 medium carrots)

½ cup roughly chopped toasted walnuts

FOR THE "CREAM CHEESE" FROSTING

¼ cup canned full-fat coconut milk

3 tablespoons pure maple syrup

1 teaspoon fresh lemon juice

¾ teaspoon apple cider vinegar

¼ teaspoon vanilla bean powder, or 1 teaspoon pure vanilla extract

⅛ teaspoon kosher salt

WALNUT CARROT CAKE WITH "CREAM CHEESE" FROSTING

PALEO • GRAIN-FREE • VEGAN • GLUTEN-FREE • DAIRY-FREE

This walnut carrot cake is a bit cakey, a little bit chewy, and laced with warm cinnamon and crunchy walnuts. It's a snack cake—not too fancy, perfect for serving during brunch or packing in a lunch box. I use cashew butter as the base because I love the rich, buttery flavor, but almond or even pecan butter would be great here too. And the frosting: It has just the right combination of lemon juice and apple cider vinegar to create a flavor that totally mimics real cream cheese frosting.

....

BEFORE you begin, soak the cashews for the frosting. Put the cashews in a large bowl and add enough water to cover by 1 or 2 inches. I prefer to use filtered water but tap water is also fine. Let the cashews soak for at least 4 hours on the countertop. If soaking longer, refrigerate for up to 12 hours. If you don't have time for the longer soak, cover the cashews with boiling water and let them soak for 1 hour. This speeds up the process although the nuts won't be as creamy as after a longer soak. Drain and rinse the cashews before using.

PREHEAT the oven to 350°F. Line an 8×8-inch baking pan with parchment paper and grease with coconut oil.

FOR THE CAKE: In a large mixing bowl, stir together the nut butter, coconut sugar, coconut oil, applesauce, and vanilla extract until smooth and well mixed. Stir in the almond flour, coconut flour, baking powder, cinnamon, and salt. Fold in the grated carrots and toasted walnuts.

SPREAD evenly in the prepared pan. Bake for 22 to 24 minutes, until lightly browned and a toothpick inserted near the center comes out clean. Cool completely in the pan set on a wire rack before topping with frosting.

FOR THE FROSTING: Drain and rinse the cashews. In a high-powered blender or the bowl of a food processor fitted with the metal blade, blend the drained cashews, coconut milk, maple syrup, lemon juice, vinegar, vanilla, and salt. Blend for 3 to 5 minutes, scraping down the sides of the blender or bowl as necessary, until the frosting is completely smooth and creamy. Taste and adjust the sweetness with a little more maple syrup, if desired.

SPREAD the frosting over the top of the cooled cake and refrigerate for at least 1 hour before cutting.

ONCE chilled, cut into 16 squares. Refrigerate in an airtight container for up to 1 week, or freeze for up to 6 months.

Tip

For the best flavor, grate fresh carrots for the cake. Don't use the pre-shredded carrots sold in the supermarket.

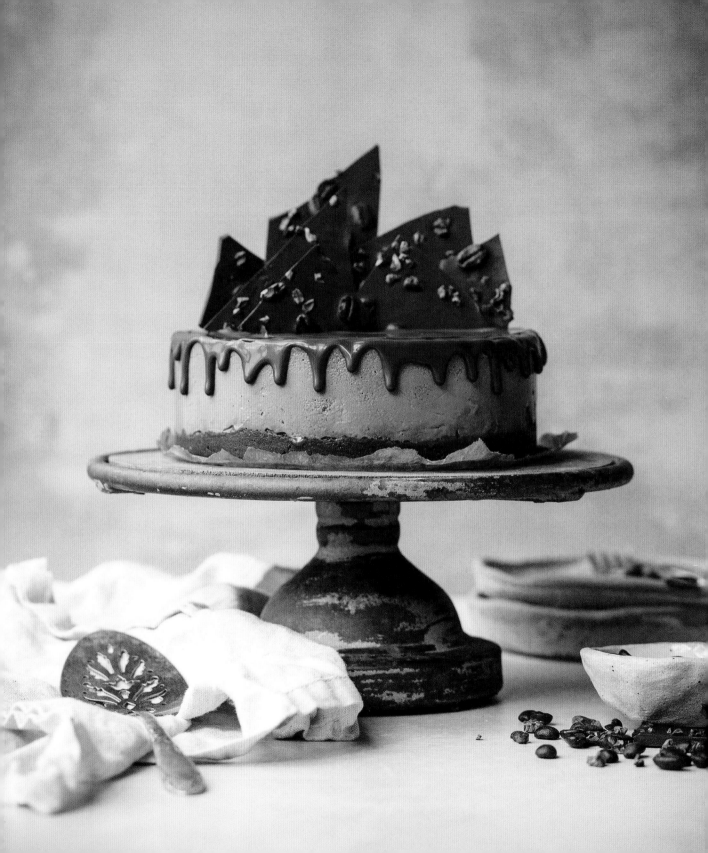

MOCHA CHIP CHEESECAKE

PALEO • GRAIN-FREE • VEGAN • NO-BAKE • GLUTEN-FREE • DAIRY-FREE

I've always been a big fan of coffee-flavored desserts. Even in the times I've banished coffee from my diet for health reasons, I've sought out coffee-flavored things to satisfy that fix. Growing up, the java chip Frappuccino from everyone's neighborhood coffee shop was my favorite thing to sip on after school. This mocha chip cheesecake is my go at re-creating those flavors. A chocolate crust serves as a firm, chocolate cookie–like base for a creamy, chocolate chip–studded mocha filling. The whole thing is topped off with a luscious chocolate ganache and shards of coffee bean–studded chocolate bark (a dessert in its own right).

BEFORE you begin, soak the cashews for the filling. Put the cashews in a large bowl and add enough water to cover by 1 or 2 inches. I prefer to use filtered water but tap water is also fine. Let the cashews soak for at least 4 hours on the countertop. If soaking longer, refrigerate for up to 12 hours. If you don't have time for the longer soak, cover the cashews with boiling water and let soak for 1 hour. This speeds up the process although the nuts won't be as creamy as after a longer soak. Drain and rinse the cashews before using.

FOR THE BARK: Line a baking sheet with parchment paper. Put the chocolate in a microwave-safe bowl and microwave for 1 minute. Stir and then microwave for another 30 seconds (you may have to do this again). Stir until melted and fluid. Spread the chocolate on the parchment paper and sprinkle with the cacao nibs and coffee beans. Refrigerate or freeze to firm up until hard, 10 to 20 minutes. Lift the chocolate from the parchment and break it into large shards. Set the bark aside at cool room temperature or in the refrigerator while preparing the cheesecake.

FOR THE CRUST: Line the bottom of a 6-inch springform pan with parchment paper and lightly grease with coconut oil. Alternatively, you can use an 8-inch square baking pan.

Prep time: 30 minutes

Chill time: 3 hours 15 minutes

Total time: 3¾ hours (plus soaking the cashews)

Yield: 10 servings

2 cups (240g) raw cashews

FOR THE COFFEE BEAN BARK

3 ounces bittersweet chocolate, chopped or in chips (about 6 tablespoons)

1 tablespoon cacao nibs

1 tablespoon whole coffee or espresso beans

FOR THE CHOCOLATE CRUST

1¼ cups (120g) blanched almond flour

¼ cup (24g) cacao powder

3 tablespoons coconut oil, melted

2 tablespoons pure maple syrup

¼ teaspoon kosher salt

FOR THE CHEESECAKE FILLING

½ cup canned full-fat coconut milk

3 tablespoons cacao butter or refined coconut oil, melted

⅓ cup pure maple syrup

⅓ cup cacao powder

2 teaspoons instant espresso powder

1 teaspoon pure vanilla extract

½ teaspoon kosher salt

2 ounces (about ⅓ cup) mini chocolate chips or cacao nibs

CONTINUES

FOR THE GANACHE

3 ounces bittersweet chocolate, chopped or in chips (about 6 tablespoons)

⅓ cup canned full-fat coconut milk

COMBINE all the crust ingredients in a mixing bowl and stir until the dough comes together. Press evenly over the bottom of the prepared pan. Refrigerate while making the filling.

FOR THE FILLING: Drain and rinse the cashews. Shake them to remove excess water. In a high-powered blender (I use a Vitamix, but most powerful blenders should do the job) or the bowl of a food processor fitted with the metal blade, combine the drained cashews, coconut milk, cacao butter, maple syrup, cacao powder, espresso powder, vanilla, and salt. Blend for 2 to 4 minutes, until the filling is silky smooth and super creamy. Stir in the chocolate chips.

POUR the filling into the prepared pan and smooth it over the crust. Tap the pan hard against the counter a few times to release any air bubbles. Freeze for at least 3 hours or until completely firm, or refrigerate for at least 6 hours until firm.

WHEN you're ready to serve, release the side of the springform pan. The cheesecake will be resting on the bottom of the springform and it will be easy to slice.

FOR THE GANACHE: Put the chopped chocolate in a small bowl. Heat the coconut milk in a saucepan or microwave until simmering. Pour over the chocolate and let the mixture stand for 3 minutes, then whisk until smooth.

SPREAD the ganache over the top of the cheesecake, letting it drip down the sides as desired. Garnish with the coffee bean bark.

STORE the cheesecake in the refrigerator for up to 5 days or the freezer for up to 2 months. If frozen, let the cake thaw at room temperature for 10 to 15 minutes before serving.

VANILLA BUNDT CAKE WITH BLOOD ORANGE GLAZE

GRAIN-FREE • PALEO • GLUTEN-FREE • DAIRY-FREE

I believe that citrus is winter's gift to us—amid all the greens at the farmers' market, I head to the tables of citrus, their gradient of oranges and pinks halved to show their glimmering, succulent insides. I'm always drawn right toward the deep red of the blood oranges. They look unassuming on the outside, but when you cut into one, it's like unearthing a glimmering sapphire—one you can eat. The blood oranges naturally tint the coconut butter-based glaze a beautiful pink color, which pairs perfectly with the rich pound cake-like texture of the vanilla Bundt cake. Add some dried blood orange slices (see Tip) and you have a stunner of a dessert that tastes as good as it looks.

PREHEAT the oven to 350°F. Grease an 8- or 9-inch Bundt pan with coconut oil; make sure to grease the center tube.

FOR THE CAKE: In a large mixing bowl, whisk the almond flour with the tapioca flour, coconut sugar, baking powder, baking soda, salt, and vanilla bean powder.

IN a separate mixing bowl, whisk together the applesauce, milk, coconut oil, eggs, and vanilla extract.

POUR the wet ingredients into the mixing bowl with the dry ingredients and stir until combined. Pour the batter into the prepared pan and use a spatula to make the top as smooth as possible.

BAKE for 30 to 35 minutes, until a toothpick inserted near the center of the cake comes out clean and the cake springs back when gently pressed. Let the cake cool completely before removing it from the pan. Invert the cake pan onto a wire rack to remove the cake. Set the wire rack and the cake on a baking sheet or large piece of parchment paper.

CONTINUES

Prep time: 15 minutes
Bake time: 30 minutes
Total time: 45 minutes
Yield: about 24 slices

FOR THE CAKE
3 cups (288g) blanched almond flour

¾ cup (85g) tapioca flour

⅔ cup (96g) coconut sugar

2 teaspoons baking powder

1 teaspoon baking soda

¾ teaspoon kosher salt

¾ teaspoon vanilla bean powder

½ cup (122g) unsweetened applesauce, at room temperature

⅔ cup dairy-free milk, such as unsweetened almond milk, warmed slightly

⅓ cup (67g) refined coconut oil, melted and cooled

3 large eggs, at room temperature

1 teaspoon pure vanilla extract

FOR THE BLOOD ORANGE GLAZE
1 cup blood orange juice

¼ cup raw honey

½ cup coconut butter

Tip

To make dried orange slices, rinse an orange with cool water and then slice it very thin—I like using a mandoline for this. Spread the slices on a baking sheet lined with parchment paper and bake at 200°F for 2 hours, or until dried.

FOR THE GLAZE: Heat the blood orange juice and honey in a small saucepan. Bring to a boil and let it boil for about 5 minutes, until the glaze is reduced by half. Add the coconut butter and whisk to combine. Let the glaze cool and thicken slightly.

POUR the glaze over the cooled cake. Any excess will drip onto the baking sheet or parchment. Let the cake sit for at least 15 minutes to give the glaze time to firm up a little before serving.

STORE the cake at room temperature, preferably under a cake dome or covered with plastic wrap, for up to 2 days, or in an airtight container in the refrigerator for up to 1 week.

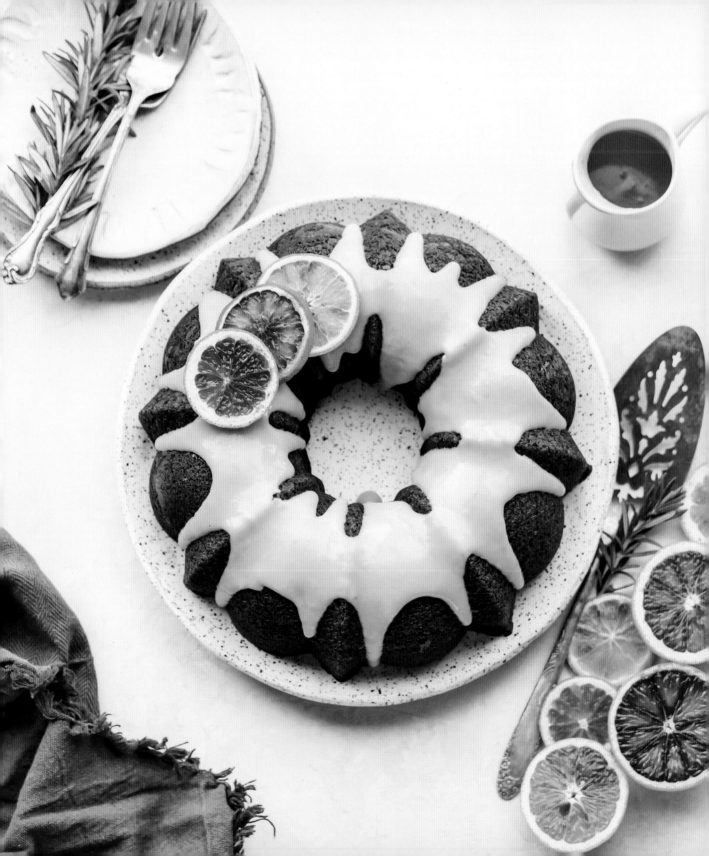

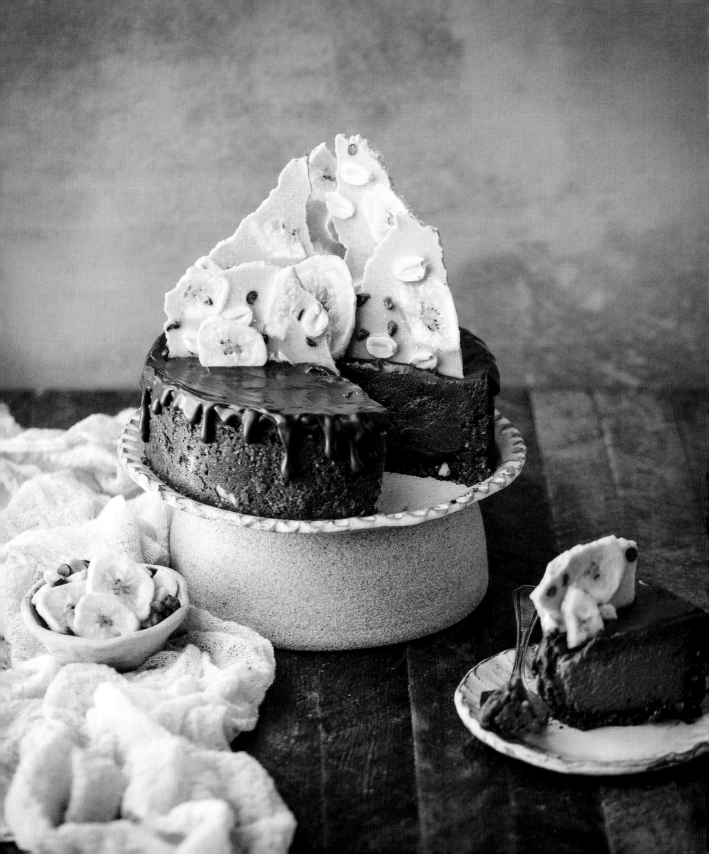

CHOCOLATE, PEANUT BUTTER, AND BANANA CHEESECAKE

GRAIN-FREE • VEGAN • NO-BAKE • GLUTEN-FREE • DAIRY-FREE

What makes a chocolate-PB-banana cheesecake even better? A crispy chocolate peanut crust to encase it, chocolate ganache to drape over the top and drip down the sides, and a simple peanut butter bark to garnish, which makes it extra beautiful. The filling uses fresh bananas in addition to soaked cashews, which makes a cake that is creamy and decadent, yet only barely sweetened with maple syrup—the ripe bananas help with a lot of the sweetening. I love the look of the peanut butter bark on top, but it's totally optional! The chocolate ganache alone is beautiful in and of itself, and you can always garnish with banana chips and peanuts for a bit of extra pizazz. Enjoy!

BEFORE you begin, soak the cashews for the filling. Put the cashews in a large bowl and add enough water to cover by 1 or 2 inches. I prefer to use filtered water but tap water is also fine. Let the cashews soak for at least 4 hours on the countertop. If soaking longer, refrigerate for up to 12 hours. If you don't have time for the longer soak, cover the cashews with boiling water and let them soak for 1 hour. This speeds up the process although the nuts won't be as creamy as after a longer soak. Drain and rinse the cashews before using.

GREASE a 6-inch springform pan with coconut oil, or line a 6-inch cake pan with strips of parchment paper for easy removal. Alternatively, you could use an 8-inch square baking pan.

FOR THE CRUST: Put all the crust ingredients in the bowl of a food processor fitted with the metal blade or a high-powered blender (I use a Vitamix). Blend until the ingredients comes together in a sticky dough with small bits of peanuts remaining. Don't overprocess, or it will turn into nut butter!

PRESS the dough evenly over the bottom and up the sides of the prepared pan.

Prep time: 30 minutes

Chill time: 3 hours

Total time: 3½ hours (plus soaking the cashews)

Yield: 8 slices

1½ cups (180g) raw cashews

FOR THE CRUST

¾ cup (72g) blanched almond flour

½ cup (57g) unsalted roasted peanuts

¼ cup (24g) cacao powder

2 tablespoons (25g) refined coconut oil, melted

2 tablespoons (32g) creamy peanut butter

2 tablespoons (42g) pure maple syrup

¼ teaspoon kosher salt

FOR THE CHEESECAKE FILLING

2 ripe bananas

¼ cup refined coconut oil

¼ cup cacao powder

3 tablespoons pure maple syrup

1½ teaspoons pure vanilla extract

½ teaspoon kosher salt

FOR THE GANACHE

3 ounces (about 6 tablespoons) bittersweet chocolate (I use 72 percent cacao), chopped

½ cup canned full-fat coconut milk

FOR THE OPTIONAL BARK

2 ounces cacao butter

¼ cup creamy peanut butter

2 tablespoons each banana chips, peanuts, and chocolate chips

CONTINUES

89

FOR THE FILLING: Drain and rinse the cashews. In the same food processor or blender (no need to wash between), combine the soaked cashews and the remaining filling ingredients and blend until the filling is silky smooth and creamy, about 2 minutes. Scrape down the sides of the bowl or blender as necessary. Taste the mixture and adjust the flavors as desired. It might need a little more maple syrup, vanilla, or cacao, to suit your taste.

POUR the filling into the prepared pan over the crust. Smooth out the top and tap the pan hard against the counter a few times to release any air bubbles. Freeze for at least 3 hours or until completely firm before decorating with the ganache.

FOR THE GANACHE: Put the chopped chocolate in a bowl. Warm the coconut milk in a saucepan until just simmering and pour over the chocolate. You can also warm the coconut milk in the microwave for 30 seconds. Make sure all the chocolate is covered by coconut milk and let the ganache stand for about 2 minutes. Stir until smooth and the chocolate melts. Spread the ganache over the cheesecake.

FOR THE BARK: Line a baking sheet with parchment paper. Microwave the cacao butter in a microwave-safe bowl for 1 minute. Stir, then microwave for another 30 seconds. Stir until melted. Add the peanut butter. Spread the mixture onto the parchment paper and sprinkle with your favorite combination of banana chips, peanuts, and chocolate chips. Refrigerate or freeze the bark until it hardens, about 10 minutes. Break into shards and arrange on the cake as desired.

SERVE immediately or freeze until ready to serve. If the cheesecake is frozen, let it thaw at room temperature for 10 to 15 minutes before slicing. To make it easy to slice, run the knife under hot water to warm it up and dry it before cutting the cheesecake with the still-hot knife. Store the cheesecake tightly wrapped in the freezer for up to 3 months.

APPLE SPICE LAYER CAKE

PALEO • GRAIN-FREE • GLUTEN-FREE • DAIRY-FREE

Skip the apple pie at Thanksgiving this year and let this apple spice cake be the star of the show! The tender, incredibly moist cake is full of sautéed apple pieces and flavored with cinnamon and nutmeg for warmth in every bite. The frosting, made with a base of soaked cashews, has cinnamon and vanilla laced through it to amplify those flavors in the cake. A flood of caramel sauce on the top makes it even more decadent. And for a true showstopper, top the cake with caramel apples—made simply with small apples dipped in the caramel sauce. The instructions below detail making a traditional two-layer cake, but I also love using three 6-inch pans to make a smaller three-layer cake for maximum impressiveness. However you stack it, this one will be devoured quickly!

Prep time: 45 minutes
Bake time: 30 minutes
Chilling time: 1 hour
Total time: 2¼ hours (plus soaking the cashews)
Yield: about 10 slices

3 cups (360g) raw cashews

FOR THE SAUTÉED APPLES
1 teaspoon refined coconut oil
2 medium apples, peeled and cut into ⅛-inch dice
2 tablespoons coconut sugar
¼ teaspoon ground cinnamon

FOR THE APPLE SPICE CAKE
3 cups (288g) blanched almond flour
⅔ cup (76g) tapioca flour
2¼ teaspoons ground cinnamon
1 teaspoon baking soda
1 teaspoon baking powder
1 teaspoon kosher salt
½ teaspoon ground nutmeg
1⅓ cups (192g) coconut sugar
⅔ cup (162g) unsweetened applesauce
½ cup dairy-free milk, such as unsweetened almond milk, warmed slightly
⅓ cup (67g) refined coconut oil, melted and cooled
2 teaspoons pure vanilla extract
2 teaspoons apple cider vinegar
4 large eggs, at room temperature

BEFORE you begin, soak the cashews for the frosting. Put the cashews in a large bowl and add enough water to cover by 1 or 2 inches. I prefer to use filtered water but tap water is also fine. Let the cashews soak for at least 4 hours on the countertop. If soaking longer, refrigerate for up to 12 hours. If you don't have time for the longer soak, cover the cashews with boiling water and let them soak for 1 hour. This speeds up the process although the nuts won't be as creamy as after a longer soak. Drain and rinse the cashews before using.

FOR THE SAUTÉED APPLES: In a small saucepan or sauté pan, melt the coconut oil over medium heat. Add the diced apples, coconut sugar, and cinnamon. Cook for a few minutes, stirring occasionally, until the sugar has melted and formed a caramel-like sauce on the apples. Remove from the heat and let cool completely.

FOR THE CAKE: Preheat the oven to 350°F; line two 8-inch round or three 6-inch round cake pans with parchment paper and grease with coconut oil.

IN a large mixing bowl, whisk the almond flour with the tapioca flour, cinnamon, baking soda, baking powder, salt, and nutmeg.

CONTINUES

FOR THE FROSTING

½ cup canned coconut cream

½ cup refined coconut oil, melted

½ cup pure maple syrup

2 teaspoons vanilla extract

1½ teaspoons ground cinnamon

¼ teaspoon vanilla bean powder

FOR OPTIONAL GARNISH

Salted Caramel Sauce (page 270)

Small apples

IN a separate mixing bowl, stir together the coconut sugar, applesauce, milk, coconut oil, vanilla, vinegar, and eggs.

POUR the wet ingredients into the dry ingredients and stir until combined. Fold in the cooled sautéed apples.

DIVIDE the batter evenly between the cake pans. Bake for 25 to 30 minutes, depending on the size of the pans, or until a toothpick inserted in the center comes out clean and the cakes spring back when gently pressed. Let the layers cool completely before removing them from the pan and frosting.

FOR THE FROSTING: In a high-powered blender (I use my Vitamix) or the bowl of a food processor fitted with the metal blade, blend the soaked cashews until they are smooth and creamy, using the tamper to keep them moving in the blender. Scrape down the sides of the food processor. Add the rest of the frosting ingredients and blend for 3 to 5 minutes, until completely smooth and creamy.

REFRIGERATE for 1 hour, then whisk by hand, or whip for about 30 seconds in a stand mixer with the whisk attachment, to fluff it up.

TO ASSEMBLE: If the layers are domed in the center, trim the tops to make them level. Put one cooled cake layer, trimmed side up, on a cake stand (or whatever you'd like to serve it on). Top with a portion of the frosting and spread evenly with an offset spatula.

TOP with the second cake layer and more frosting. If you have a third layer, place it on top and spread the remaining frosting across the top and down the sides of the cake, spreading evenly.

KEEP as is, or garnish with Salted Caramel Sauce and small apples dipped in the caramel sauce. Store covered in the refrigerator for up to 5 days.

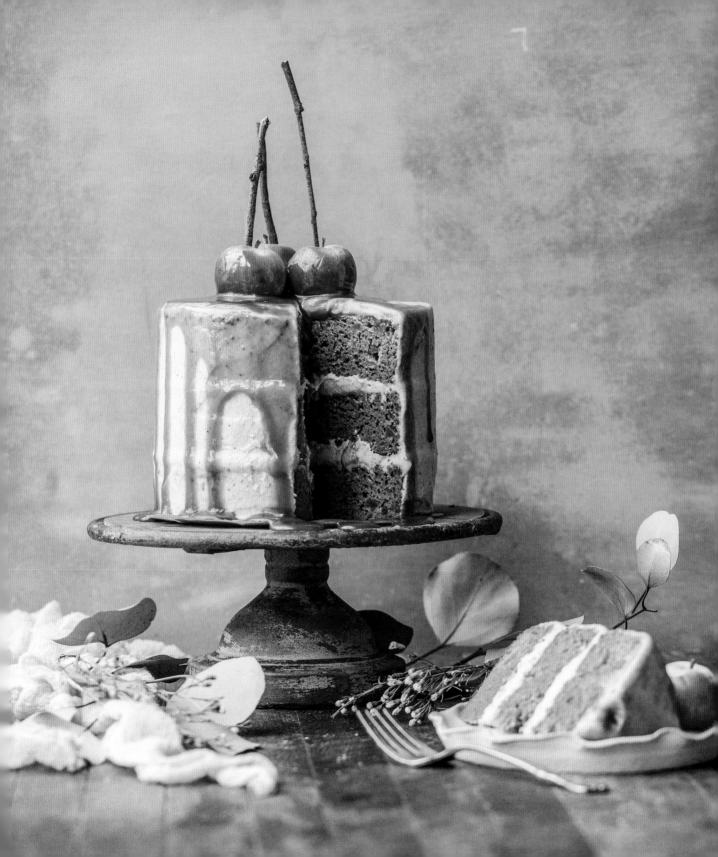

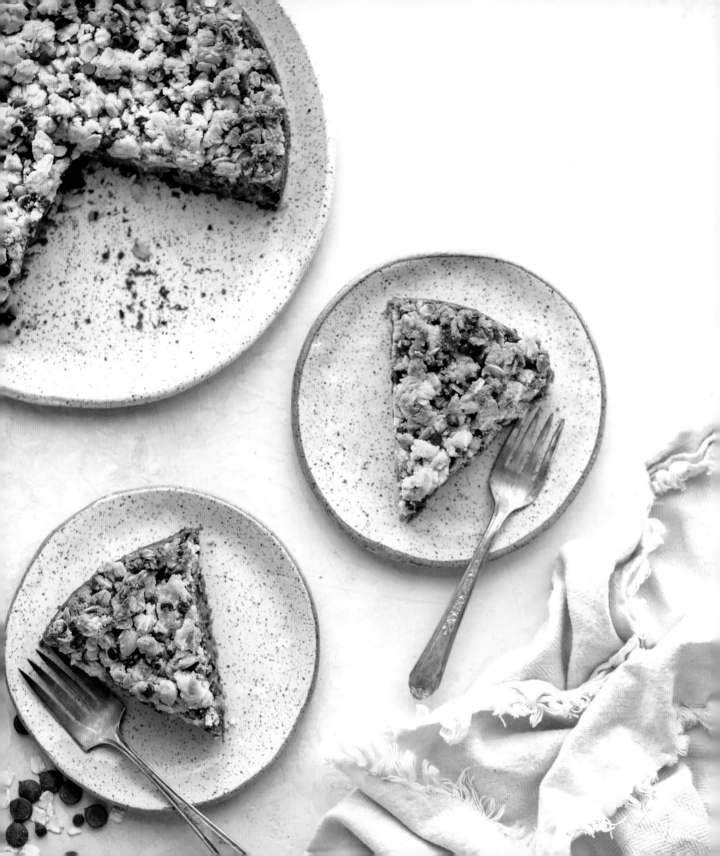

OATMEAL–CHOCOLATE CHIP CRUMB CAKE

VEGAN • GLUTEN-FREE • DAIRY-FREE

This crumb cake reminds me of a cake I made all the time back in high school—certainly not gluten-free and vegan in those days. I've always been a big fan of oatmeal–chocolate chip cookies, and this is essentially those, but in *cake* form. It can be served as a decadent breakfast or brunch option or topped with some coconut whipped cream or dairy-free ice cream for a delicious dessert. Oh, and do your best not to eat all the crumble off the top before you serve it— it'll be a test of wills!

PREHEAT the oven to 350°F. Line an 8-inch round cake pan or springform pan with parchment paper and grease the paper with coconut oil.

FOR THE CAKE: Combine the almond milk and vinegar in a bowl and set aside for 5 or 10 minutes to give the milk time to curdle.

MEANWHILE, whisk the almond flour with the rolled oats, tapioca flour, coconut sugar, baking powder, baking soda, salt, and cinnamon in a large bowl, making sure to get all the clumps out.

ADD the melted coconut oil and flax eggs to the curdled milk and whisk until smooth. Add the wet mixture to the dry ingredients and stir until smooth and the dry ingredients are coated with the wet. Fold in the chocolate chips. Scrape the batter into the prepared pan, smoothing it with a rubber spatula or the back of a spoon.

FOR THE CRUMBLE: Stir the almond flour with the coconut flour, rolled oats, salt, and coconut oil. Add the maple syrup and stir until the dry ingredients are completely moistened. Finally, mix in the chocolate chips. Scatter the crumble evenly over the batter.

BAKE the cake until golden brown and a toothpick inserted into the center comes out clean, 45 to 55 minutes. If necessary, cover the cake with foil after about 20 minutes to keep the crumb topping from getting too brown.

Prep time: 15 minutes
Bake time: 45 minutes
Total time: 1 hour
Yield: 10 slices

FOR THE CAKE

- ¾ cup unsweetened almond milk or other dairy-free milk, at room temperature
- 1 tablespoon apple cider vinegar
- 1⅔ cups (160g) blanched almond flour
- 1 cup (96g) gluten-free rolled oats
- ½ cup (57g) tapioca flour
- ½ cup (72g) coconut sugar
- 2 teaspoons baking powder
- 1 teaspoon baking soda
- 1 teaspoon kosher salt
- ¾ teaspoon ground cinnamon
- ⅓ cup (67g) refined coconut oil, melted
- 2 flax eggs (see Tips)
- 2 ounces (about ⅓ cup) bittersweet chocolate chips

FOR THE CRUMBLE

- ¾ cup (75g) blanched almond flour
- 2 tablespoons coconut flour
- ½ cup (48g) gluten-free rolled oats
- ¼ teaspoon sea salt
- 3 tablespoons (37g) refined coconut oil, softened (see Tips)
- 3 tablespoons (63g) pure maple syrup
- 1½ ounces (about ¼ cup) mini chocolate chips

CONTINUES

SET the cake in the pan on a wire rack and let sit until completely cool. Serve the cake or store in an airtight container at room temperature for up to 3 days, or in the refrigerator for up to 1 week. The cake can also be frozen for up to 3 months. I love refrigerated slices warmed in the microwave for about 20 seconds to melt the chocolate!

Tips

- To make 2 flax eggs, mix 2 tablespoons ground flax seed with 5 tablespoons water and whisk well. Set aside for about 10 minutes to give the mixture time to gel.
- The coconut oil should be the texture of softened butter. If it melts to a liquid because the kitchen is too warm, refrigerate for 15 to 20 minutes until it solidifies.

COCONUT CUPCAKES WITH COCONUT FROSTING

PALEO • GRAIN-FREE • NUT-FREE • GLUTEN-FREE • DAIRY-FREE

As soon as I bit into one of these coconut cupcakes, they became a quick favorite: moist, rich, and full of coconut flavor, with some texture from the coconut mixed into the batter and frosting. When I was a kid, my mom would make a coconut cupcake similar to this, with loads of coconut in the cake, in the frosting, and more on top. These bring back all sorts of memories of devouring those coconut cupcakes, fresh from the oven with melting icing, in the kitchen with my mom.

BEFORE you begin, soak the cashews for the frosting. Put the cashews in a large bowl and add enough water to cover by 1 or 2 inches. I prefer to use filtered water but tap water is also fine. Let the cashews soak for at least 4 hours on the countertop. If soaking longer, refrigerate for up to 12 hours. If you don't have time for the longer soak, cover the cashews with boiling water and let them soak for 1 hour. This speeds up the process although the nuts won't be as creamy as after a longer soak. Drain and rinse the cashews before using.

FOR THE CUPCAKES: Preheat the oven to 350°F. Line 10 cups of a 12-cup cupcake tin with paper liners or grease lightly with coconut oil.

IN a mixing bowl, whisk together the shredded coconut, coconut flour, baking powder, baking soda, salt, and coconut sugar.

IN a separate bowl or large liquid measuring cup, stir together the coconut milk, coconut oil, maple syrup, eggs, and vanilla extract.

POUR the liquid ingredients into the dry ingredients and stir to combine. Let the batter sit for about 3 minutes to let the coconut flour absorb some of the liquid.

Prep time: 20 minutes
Bake time: 22 minutes
Chill time: 1 hour
Total time: 1 hour 42 minutes (plus soaking the cashews)
Yield: 10 cupcakes

1 cup (120g) raw cashews

FOR THE CUPCAKES
1 cup (80g) unsweetened finely shredded coconut
½ cup (64g) coconut flour
½ teaspoon baking powder
½ teaspoon baking soda
¼ teaspoon kosher salt
⅓ cup (48g) coconut sugar
½ cup canned full-fat coconut milk
⅓ cup (67g) virgin coconut oil, melted
⅓ cup (111g) pure maple syrup
3 large eggs, at room temperature
1½ teaspoons pure vanilla extract

FOR THE FROSTING
½ cup unsweetened shredded coconut, plus more for garnish
⅓ cup coconut butter, melted
⅓ cup canned coconut cream
2 tablespoons refined coconut oil, melted
¼ cup pure maple syrup
½ teaspoon pure vanilla extract
½ teaspoon pure almond extract
⅛ teaspoon sea salt

DIVIDE the batter among the cupcake cups, filling each about two-thirds full. If your cupcake pan has 12 cups, pour a little water in the empty cups so they won't be empty during baking.

BAKE for 22 to 25 minutes, until a toothpick inserted in the center of a cupcake comes out clean and the tops of the cupcakes bounce back when touched lightly with a finger. Let the cupcakes cool for 10 minutes in the pan before removing to a wire rack to cool completely.

FOR THE FROSTING: Drain the cashews and shake gently in the colander to rid them of excess water.

SPREAD the coconut in a large skillet (add a little extra coconut if you want it for garnish). Set the pan over moderate heat and cook, stirring gently, until the coconut browns and toasts, 3 to 5 minutes. When the edges of the coconut shreds turn light brown and aromatic, remove the coconut from the pan and spread it on a plate to cool.

IN a large mixing bowl, stir together the coconut butter and coconut cream until smooth. Transfer to a high-powered blender (I use a Vitamix) or the bowl of a food processor fitted with a metal blade. Add the drained cashews, coconut oil, maple syrup, vanilla extract, almond extract, and salt and mix for 3 to 5 minutes, until smooth and creamy. Add the coconut and stir or pulse to mix.

IF you like the consistency of the frosting as it is now, spread it over the tops of the cooled cupcakes. If you would like to pipe the frosting, transfer to a metal bowl and refrigerate for 1 hour, whisking every 20 minutes, until it's thick enough to pipe on top of the cupcakes.

TRANSFER the frosting to a piping bag fitted with a large star piping tip or a zippered plastic bag with the corner snipped off and pipe the frosting on the cupcakes.

AFTER frosting the cupcakes, garnish each with a sprinkle of toasted coconut.

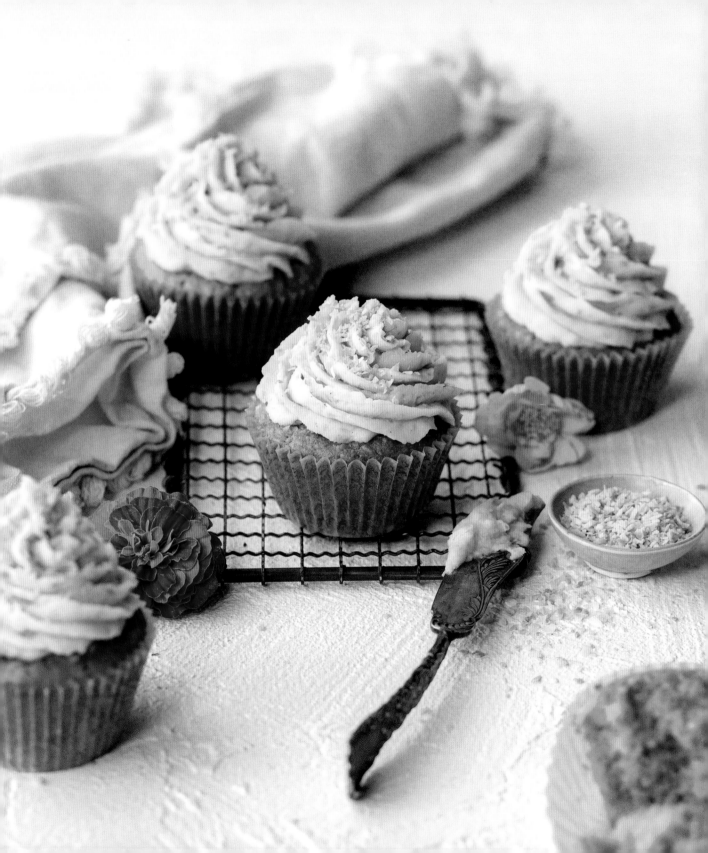

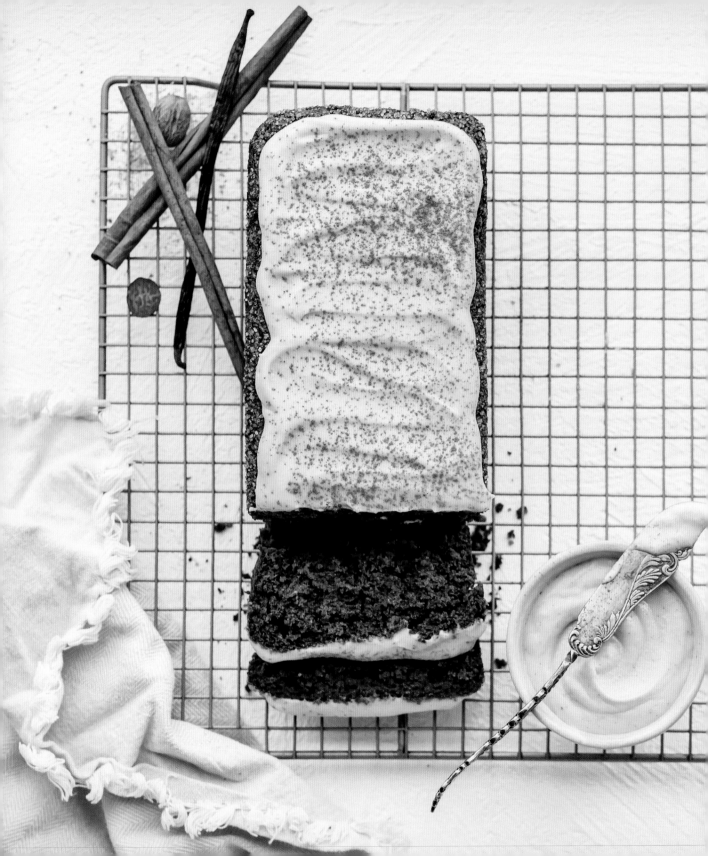

GINGERBREAD LOAF WITH VANILLA "CREAM CHEESE" FROSTING

VEGAN • GLUTEN-FREE • DAIRY-FREE

This recipe took me more tries to nail than I'm willing to admit, but to be real, it was certainly not the worst thing in the world to have a few less-than-perfect gingerbread loaves hanging around. Spiced with cinnamon, ginger, nutmeg, and cloves, this loaf will make your house smell like the holidays no matter the season. I sprinkle some raw turbinado sugar on top of the batter, which adds the most delicious layer of crunchy sugar crust. You can leave it there or go the extra mile and spread tangy vanilla "cream cheese"–style frosting on top. With or without frosting, you'll be sneaking slivers of this spicy loaf all day long.

BEFORE you begin, soak the cashews for the frosting. Put the cashews in a large bowl and add enough water to cover by 1 or 2 inches. I prefer to use filtered water but tap water is also fine. Let the cashews soak for at least 4 hours on the countertop. If soaking longer, refrigerate for up to 12 hours. If you don't have time for the longer soak, cover the cashews with boiling water and let them soak for 1 hour. This speeds up the process although the nuts won't be as creamy as after a longer soak. Drain and rinse the cashews before using.

PREHEAT the oven to 350°F. Grease an 8½ × 4½-inch loaf pan with coconut oil or line it with parchment paper, or do both. You could also use a 9 × 5-inch loaf pan, though the loaf will be thinner.

FOR THE LOAF: In a small bowl or liquid measuring cup, combine the milk and vinegar. Set aside for 5 to 10 minutes to give the milk time to curdle.

IN a mixing bowl, stir together the curdled milk, coconut sugar, pumpkin puree, nut butter, coconut oil, molasses, ground flax seed, and vanilla extract. Whisk or stir to combine.

Prep time: 20 minutes

Bake time: 50 minutes

Total time: 1 hour 10 minutes (plus soaking the cashews)

Yield: about 10 slices

1 cup (120g) raw cashews

FOR THE GINGERBREAD LOAF

¼ cup unsweetened almond milk or other dairy-free milk

1 tablespoon apple cider vinegar

¾ cup (108g) coconut sugar

½ cup (122g) pure pumpkin puree

⅓ cup (85g) almond or cashew butter (see Tips)

2 tablespoons virgin coconut oil, melted

2 tablespoons organic molasses

2 tablespoons ground flax seed

1 teaspoon pure vanilla extract

1¼ cups (120g) blanched almond flour

1 cup (120g) gluten-free oat flour (see Tips)

1 teaspoon baking soda

1 teaspoon baking powder

2 teaspoons ground cinnamon

1½ teaspoons ground ginger

½ teaspoon nutmeg

½ teaspoon sea salt

¼ teaspoon ground cloves

2 tablespoons raw turbinado sugar (optional)

CONTINUES

FOR THE FROSTING

¼ cup canned full-fat
   coconut milk

3 tablespoons pure maple syrup

1 tablespoon refined coconut oil,
   melted

¾ teaspoon fresh lemon juice

½ teaspoon apple cider vinegar

¼ teaspoon vanilla bean powder

Tips

- While I find almond and cashew butter work best here, you can use another nut or seed butter to suit your taste.
- I make my own gluten-free oat flour by grinding oats in the blender until they're finely ground to a flour-like texture, about 30 seconds.

ADD the almond flour, oat flour, baking soda, baking powder, cinnamon, ginger, nutmeg, salt, and cloves and stir until well mixed.

POUR the batter into the prepared loaf pan and smooth the top. If desired, sprinkle the top of the loaf with the raw turbinado sugar to add a little crunch. Bake for 50 minutes to 1 hour, until a knife inserted near the center comes out clean. If you're using a 9 × 5-inch loaf pan, check on the bread after 40 to 45 minutes.

LET the loaf cool in the pan for 15 minutes on a wire rack. Remove the loaf from the pan and let cool completely on the wire rack before frosting.

FOR THE FROSTING: Rinse and drain the cashews. In a high-powered blender or bowl of a food processor fitted with the metal blade, combine the drained cashews with the remaining frosting ingredients. Blend until completely smooth and creamy, about 3 minutes. Spread the frosting on top of the cooled loaf. Dust with a little cinnamon, if desired, and serve.

STORE leftovers tightly wrapped in plastic wrap, foil, or in a sealed container in the refrigerator for up to 1 week, or in the freezer for up to 6 months. If you choose not to frost the gingerbread loaf, wrap it tightly in plastic wrap or foil and keep it on the counter for up to 3 days. I like to slice it and then freeze the slices so I can grab one and heat it in the microwave whenever I want!

PALEO CHOCOLATE MELTING CAKES

PALEO • GRAIN-FREE • GLUTEN-FREE • DAIRY-FREE

A few years ago, our family went on a cruise through the Mediterranean Sea, with stops in Greece, Italy, and Spain. While of course the food we ate on shore was magnificent, there was one dessert from the trip that stood out in my mind after we disembarked: the melty chocolate lava cakes topped with a big scoop of vanilla ice cream that we ordered every night we ate dinner on board. When I got home, I re-created the dreamy chocolate melting cakes with just a few simple ingredients, adjusting some key ingredients to keep the recipe gluten-free and refined sugar–free. Nothing beats that moment when your spoon breaks through the top layer of cake into the gooey, melted chocolate center. So make sure to keep an eye on these cakes—just a few seconds too long in the oven can be the difference between a luscious, dripping chocolate center and a firmer, cakey one.

Prep time: 15 minutes
Bake time: 15 minutes
Total time: 30 minutes
Yield: 4 individual cakes

- 4 ounces (120g) bittersweet chocolate (I use 72 percent cacao; see Tips)
- ½ cup (100g) refined coconut oil or ghee (see Tips)
- 3 large eggs plus 1 large egg yolk, at room temperature
- 3 tablespoons coconut sugar
- ¼ cup (24g) blanched almond flour
- Whipped coconut cream or ice cream, for serving (optional)

PREHEAT the oven to 375°F. Lightly grease four 3-inch ramekins with coconut oil and put them on a baking sheet.

MELT the chocolate and coconut oil together in a saucepan over low heat. Once melted, remove from the heat.

IN a mixing bowl, whisk 2 of the eggs with the coconut sugar until foamy. Add the almond flour and mix well. Add the remaining egg and egg yolk and whisk to incorporate. Add the egg mixture to the melted chocolate and mix together until smooth.

DIVIDE the batter evenly among the four prepared ramekins. (If you don't want to serve right away, refrigerate the cakes until you're ready to bake.)

BAKE for about 15 minutes, until the edges are set but the center still jiggles when you gently shake the baking sheet. Start checking on the cakes after 13 minutes to ensure they don't overbake. The cakes should be soft and gooey in the center when you serve them. Serve immediately, preferably with whipped coconut cream or ice cream!

CONTINUES

Tips

- The richness of the cake is dependent on the darkness of the chocolate. If you prefer a sweeter cake, use a lighter chocolate (such as one with 60 percent cacao); but if you want a deeper, darker cake, use chocolate with a higher percentage—although I wouldn't go above 80 percent.
- To be completely dairy-free, use coconut oil. Ghee is lactose-free but still a dairy-derived product. If you don't have a problem with dairy, ½ cup (1 stick) of grass-fed butter can be used in this recipe in place of the coconut oil.

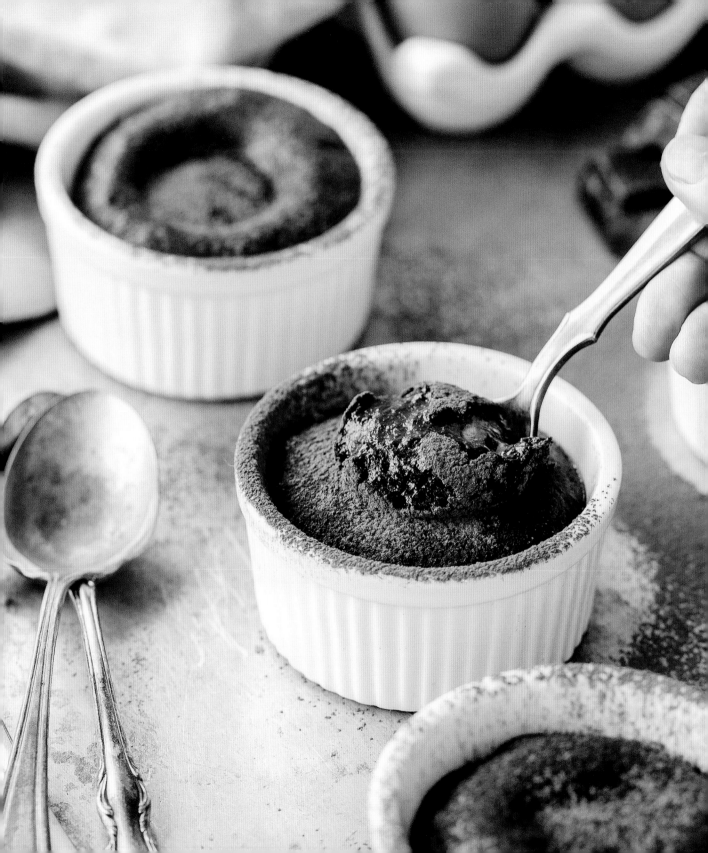

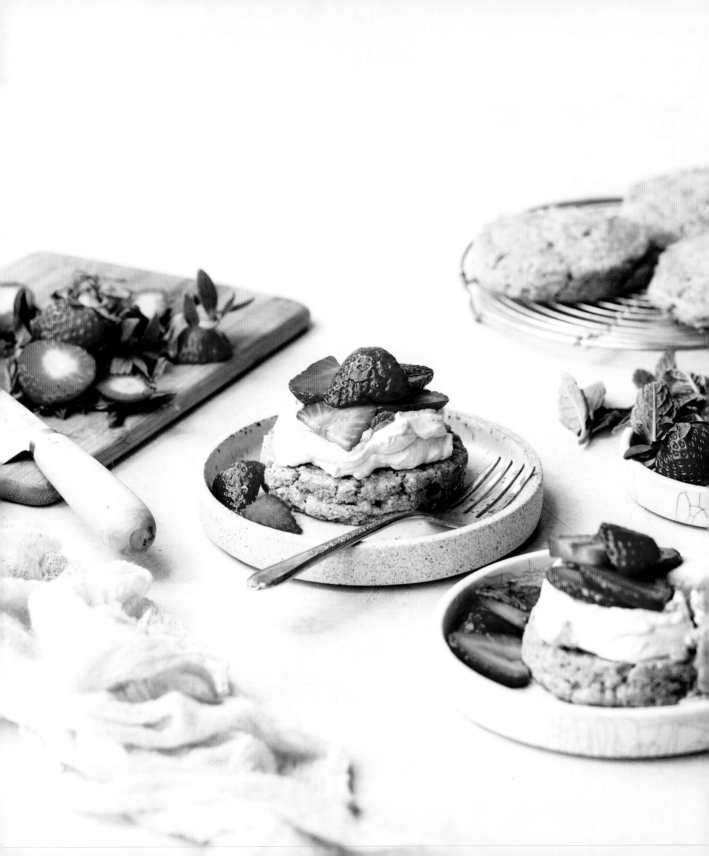

STRAWBERRY SHORTCAKES

A tender vanilla-scented shortcake dolloped with a fluff of barely sweetened coconut cream, topped with macerated strawberry slices, and scattered with freshly torn mint leaves. This is the most perfect way I can think of to celebrate the peak of strawberry season because this simple recipe highlights the red-fleshed fruit so beautifully. The shortcakes, which are somewhere between a biscuit and a scone, provide a crisp, crumbly, not-overly-sweet base for the refreshing coconut cream and, of course, those lemon-scented berries. Torn mint leaves add an herby freshness that makes this dessert irresistible.

Strawberry Shortcakes are best when they're freshly assembled, so keep the components separate until you're ready to serve.

Prep time: 40 minutes
Bake time: 25 minutes
Yield: 6 to 7 shortcakes

FOR THE BISCUITS

1¼ cups (120g) blanched almond flour

⅔ cup (80g) gluten-free oat flour

1 tablespoon baking powder

1 tablespoon coconut sugar

¼ teaspoon salt

¼ teaspoon vanilla bean powder, or ½ teaspoon vanilla extract

½ cup (100g) refined coconut oil, solid

⅓ cup (2.6 ounces) full-fat canned coconut milk, plus more to brush on the dough

1 flax egg (see Tip)

Raw turbinado sugar to sprinkle on top (optional)

FOR THE STRAWBERRIES

2 cups (1 pint) sliced fresh strawberries

1 tablespoon coconut sugar or to taste, depending on how sweet your strawberries are

Grated zest of 1 lemon

½ teaspoon vanilla extract

Leaves from 1 sprig mint, torn into bits

FOR THE CREAM

1 (13.5-ounce) can coconut cream, chilled overnight

1 tablespoon pure maple syrup

¼ teaspoon vanilla bean powder, or 1 teaspoon vanilla extract

FOR THE BISCUITS: Line a baking sheet with parchment paper and dust with oat flour.

IN a food processor or large mixing bowl, combine the almond flour, oat flour, baking powder, coconut sugar, salt, and vanilla bean powder. Pulse or whisk together.

ADD the coconut oil and pulse or use a pastry cutter or fork to work it into the dry ingredients until only small chunks of coconut oil remain—the texture should be mostly sandy.

IN a small mixing bowl, whisk together the coconut milk and flax egg. Add to the dry ingredients and stir or pulse until completely combined.

PUT the dough on the parchment paper and press it into a square about 1 inch thick. Refrigerate for 1 hour or up to 1 day, until chilled.

WHEN ready to bake, preheat the oven to 400°F.

REMOVE the dough from the refrigerator and place it on a work surface, keeping it on the parchment paper. Use a rolling pin to roll the dough out enough to flatten it and form an approximately 9-inch square. Using a 3-inch biscuit cutter, press out 6 or 7 rounds, then gather the dough scraps, reroll them, and cut out more biscuits.

CONTINUES

107

Tip

To make a flax egg, mix
1 tablespoon ground flax seed
with 2½ tablespoons water.
Whisk well and then set aside
at room temperature for
about 10 minutes to gel.

Place the rounds back on the parchment lined–baking sheet with room between each so they're not touching.

BRUSH the top of each shortcake with coconut milk and sprinkle with turbinado sugar. Bake for 20 to 25 minutes or until golden brown.

FOR THE STRAWBERRIES: While the shortcakes bake, combine the strawberries, coconut sugar, lemon zest, vanilla, and mint in a small bowl to macerate.

FOR THE CREAM: Drain the liquid from the can of coconut cream. (Keep this liquid or not; it's good in smoothies.) Transfer the cream to a mixing bowl or the bowl of a stand mixer fitted with the whisk attachment and whisk until smooth and fluffy, about 30 seconds or so. Add the maple syrup and vanilla and whisk to combine.

WHEN ready to serve, place each biscuit on a plate and top with some of the cream and macerated strawberries. Store any leftover biscuits in an airtight container at room temperature for up to 3 days. They can also be frozen if wrapped tightly and stored in an airtight container. Store any extra strawberries and cream in separate airtight containers in the refrigerator for up to 2 days.

PECAN PRALINE CHEESECAKE

PALEO · GRAIN-FREE · VEGAN · NO-BAKE · GLUTEN-FREE · DAIRY-FREE

Buttery, sweet, and chewy are the things that come to mind when I hear "pecan praline." With those words, I also usually think: butter, white sugar, heavy cream. When I was making caramel sauce and dipped a pecan into it to taste, I was hit with all the flavors of pecan pralines, without the dairy and refined sugars. This creamy cashew cheesecake brings those rich, decadent, caramel-y flavors to life. The creamy filling laced with pecan butter in the date-pecan crust is topped off with a caramel pecan sauce. This dessert is decadent and perfect for serving a crowd, because you really only need a sliver!

BEFORE you begin, soak the cashews for the filling. Put the cashews in a large bowl and add enough water to cover by 1 or 2 inches. I prefer to use filtered water but tap water is also fine. Let the cashews soak for at least 4 hours on the countertop. If soaking longer, refrigerate for up to 12 hours. If you don't have time for the longer soak, cover the cashews with boiling water and let them soak for 1 hour. This speeds up the process although the nuts won't be as creamy as after a longer soak. Drain and rinse the cashews before using.

FOR THE CARAMEL SAUCE: In a medium heavy-bottomed saucepan, bring the maple syrup, coconut sugar, and coconut milk to a boil over medium heat. As soon as the mixture boils, reduce the heat and simmer for 30 to 45 minutes, stirring frequently, until a candy thermometer reaches 234°F. Pour the sauce into a glass liquid measuring cup and set aside to cool slightly while preparing the cheesecake.

FOR THE CRUST: Grease a 6-inch springform pan with coconut oil, or line a 6-inch cake pan with strips of parchment paper for easy removal and grease well with coconut oil. Alternatively, you can use an 8-inch square baking pan.

COMBINE the roughly chopped pecans, almond flour, pitted dates, coconut oil, cinnamon, and salt in a high-powered blender

Prep time: 30 minutes
Cook time: 30 minutes
Chill time: 3 hours
Total time: 4 hours (plus soaking the cashews)
Yield: 10 slices

2 cups (240g) raw cashews

FOR THE CARAMEL SAUCE
½ cup pure maple syrup
¼ cup coconut sugar
¾ cup canned full-fat coconut milk

FOR THE DATE-PECAN CRUST
½ cup (128g) roughly chopped pecans
½ cup (48g) blanched almond flour
4 Medjool dates, pitted
1 tablespoon refined coconut oil, softened
½ teaspoon ground cinnamon
¼ teaspoon sea salt

FOR THE CHEESECAKE FILLING
½ cup canned full-fat coconut milk
¼ cup refined coconut oil, melted and cooled
2 tablespoons smooth pecan butter
2 tablespoons fresh lemon juice
¼ teaspoon vanilla bean powder
¼ teaspoon kosher salt
½ cup finely chopped pecans

CONTINUES

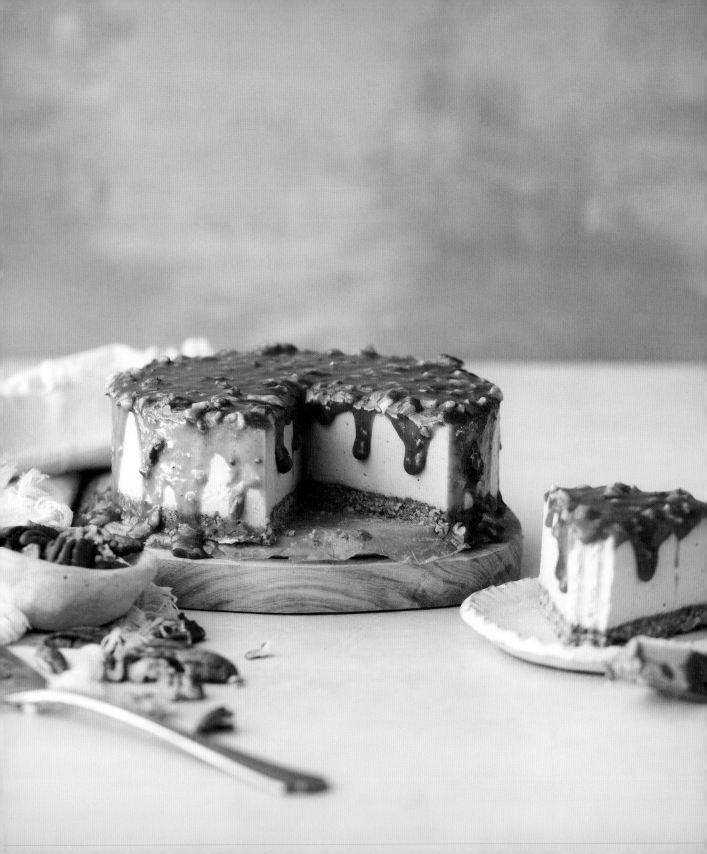

(I use a Vitamix, although most powerful blenders should work) or the bowl of a food processor fitted with the metal blade. Process until the ingredients come together in a sort of sticky dough. Don't overprocess or you will end up with nut butter. Press the dough evenly over the bottom of the prepared pan.

FOR THE FILLING: Drain and rinse the cashews. In the same food processor or high-powered blender (no need to wash between uses), combine the drained cashews, ⅓ cup of the caramel sauce, the coconut milk, coconut oil, pecan butter, lemon juice, vanilla, and salt. Blend for 2 to 4 minutes, until the mixture is silky smooth and creamy. Scrape down the sides of the blender's canister or food processor's bowl as necessary.

POUR the filling into the prepared pan over the crust. Smooth out the top and tap the pan hard against the counter a few times to release any air bubbles. Put the cheesecake in the freezer to set, at least 3 hours or until completely firm.

WHEN ready to serve, let the cheesecake thaw in the refrigerator for a few hours, or at room temperature for about 15 minutes. Stir the finely chopped pecans into the remaining caramel and pour over the cheesecake. If the caramel has cooled too much to be pourable, heat it for 15 to 30 seconds in the microwave to reliquefy.

TIGHTLY wrap and refrigerate leftovers for up to 5 days, or freeze for up to 3 months.

Prep time: 20 minutes
Bake time: 40 minutes
Total time: 1 hour
Yield: about 10 slices

FOR THE CAKE

2¼ cups (216g) blanched almond flour

⅔ cup (96g) coconut sugar

½ cup (57g) tapioca flour

⅓ cup (43g) coconut flour

2 teaspoons baking soda

1 teaspoon kosher salt

½ teaspoon ground cinnamon

3 tablespoons freshly grated orange zest plus 1 cup freshly squeezed orange juice (from 2 to 4 medium oranges)

¼ cup (50g) olive oil

¼ cup (85g) honey or pure maple syrup (see Tips)

2 flax eggs (see Tips)

2 teaspoons pure vanilla extract

FOR THE COCONUT-YOGURT FROSTING

1 cup canned coconut cream, chilled

½ cup coconut yogurt or any thick dairy-free yogurt (see Tips)

¼ teaspoon vanilla bean powder, or 1 teaspoon vanilla extract

Grated zest of 1 large orange

OPTIONAL GARNISHES

Dried orange slices

Fresh berries

Bee pollen and honey for drizzling (see Tips)

ORANGE CAKE WITH COCONUT-YOGURT FROSTING

PALEO • GRAIN-FREE • VEGAN • GLUTEN-FREE • DAIRY-FREE

This is the kind of cake that begs to be served for breakfast, is perfect for brunch get-togethers, and is also great alongside coffee or tea as a midafternoon snack. But it is also super satisfying as a dessert! The cake is tender with a beautiful orange flavor from the loads of fresh orange zest and juice. The creamy "frosting" is light and refreshing, thanks to the coconut yogurt. Coconut yogurt has a thick texture, which is recommended—a thinner yogurt could make it too runny; see the Tips. Garnish the frosted cake with fresh berries, dried orange slices, and bee pollen for a simple, stunning cake.

PREHEAT the oven to 350°F; lightly grease a 9-inch springform pan with coconut oil.

FOR THE CAKE: In a large mixing bowl, whisk the almond flour with the coconut sugar, tapioca flour, coconut flour, baking soda, salt, and cinnamon until thoroughly mixed. Form a well in the center of the dry ingredients.

IN a separate bowl, stir together the orange zest and juice, olive oil, honey, flax eggs, and vanilla extract. Pour the liquid ingredients into the well in the dry ingredients and stir to combine. Pour the batter into the prepared pan and smooth the top.

BAKE for about 40 minutes, until a toothpick inserted in the center of the cake comes out clean and the cake springs back when gently pressed with a fingertip. Set the cake in the pan on a wire rack and let cool completely. When cool, remove the cake from the pan.

FOR THE FROSTING: Place the coconut cream in a bowl or the bowl of a stand mixer fitted with the whisk attachment. Whisk until the mixture is light and fluffy. Add the coconut yogurt and vanilla and mix again. With a spoon or rubber spatula, fold the orange zest into the frosting, reserving a little for decoration, if desired.

CONTINUES

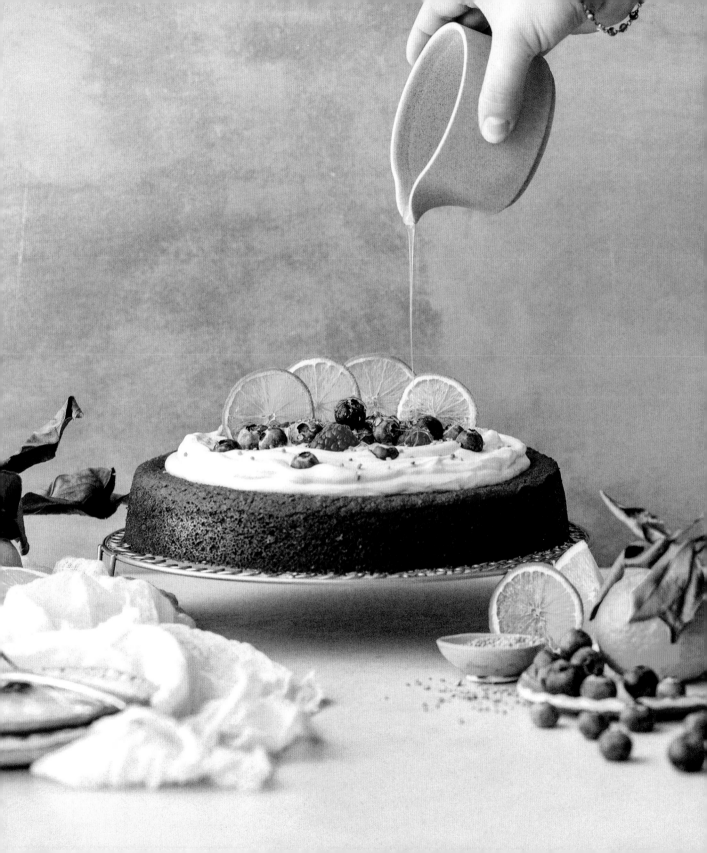

SPREAD the frosting over the cooled cake and garnish with dried orange slices, orange zest, berries, bee pollen, and honey or any combination of these garnishes, if desired.

Tips

- You can use your favorite brand of dairy-free yogurt, but keep in mind that for this recipe, the thicker the better! If your yogurt is not thick, drain about 1 cup of the thin yogurt in a fine-mesh sieve set over a bowl for 30 minutes to 1 hour, until thickened. Measure ½ cup of the thickened yogurt to use in the frosting. Or, if your yogurt is superthin, start with ¼ cup, mix, and add more if the frosting is not too runny.
- If you want to keep this vegan, use maple syrup rather than honey and don't garnish with bee pollen and honey.
- To make 2 flax eggs, whisk 2 tablespoons ground flax seed with 5 tablespoons water. Set aside for about 10 minutes to give the mixture time to gel.

NEAPOLITAN CHEESECAKE

PALEO • GRAIN-FREE • VEGAN • NO-BAKE • GLUTEN-FREE • DAIRY-FREE

Were you ever a fan of Neapolitan ice cream? When I was a kid, I loved it—but I generally dug around the strawberry and left a big gaping hole where the chocolate and vanilla were. These days I'm an equal opportunity lover of all three flavors, and they all get the chance to shine in this Neapolitan cheesecake, which is beautifully layered with chocolate, vanilla, and strawberry fillings and topped with a rich chocolate ganache. If you really want clean layers of the colors, make sure each layer is frozen (at least 30 minutes) before adding the next. If you don't mind them not being perfectly neat, you can layer them on top of each other immediately.

BEFORE you begin, soak the cashews for the filling. Put the cashews in a large bowl and add enough water to cover by 1 or 2 inches. I prefer to use filtered water but tap water is also fine. Let the cashews soak for at least 4 hours on the countertop. If soaking longer, refrigerate for up to 12 hours. If you don't have time for the longer soak, cover the cashews with boiling water and let them soak for 1 hour. This speeds up the process although the nuts won't be as creamy as with a longer soak. Drain and rinse the cashews before using.

GREASE a 6-inch springform pan with coconut oil, or line a 6-inch cake pan with strips of parchment paper for easy removal and grease well with coconut oil. Alternatively, you can use an 8-inch square baking pan.

FOR THE CRUST: Combine the almond flour, pitted dates, coconut oil, cacao powder, and salt in the bowl of a food processor fitted with the metal blade or a high-powered blender. Blend until the ingredients come together in a cohesive dough that holds together when pressed. (Don't overprocess, or the dough will turn into nut butter!) Press the crust evenly over the bottom of the prepared pan.

FOR THE FILLING: Drain and rinse the cashews. In the same food processor or high-powered blender used for the crust (no

Prep time: 30 minutes

Chill time: about 4 hours

Total time: 4½ hours (plus soaking the cashews)

Yield: 10 slices

2 cups (240g) raw cashews

FOR THE CRUST

1 cup (96g) blanched almond flour

2 Medjool dates, pitted

2 tablespoons refined coconut oil, melted

1 tablespoon cacao powder

¼ teaspoon kosher salt

FOR THE CHEESECAKE FILLING

½ cup canned full-fat coconut milk

¼ cup refined coconut oil, melted

⅓ cup pure maple syrup

2 tablespoons fresh lemon juice

1½ teaspoons pure vanilla extract, or ¾ teaspoon vanilla bean powder

4 teaspoons cacao powder

½ cup freeze-dried strawberries

FOR THE GANACHE

3 ounces (about 6 tablespoons) bittersweet chocolate (I use 72 percent cacao), chopped

⅓ cup shaken canned full-fat coconut milk

CONTINUES

need to rinse between uses), combine the drained cashews, coconut milk, coconut oil, maple syrup, lemon juice, and vanilla and blend until the filling is silky smooth and creamy, about 2 minutes. Scrape down the sides of the bowl or blender's canister as necessary.

TRANSFER two-thirds of the filling to a separate bowl (see Tip). Add the cacao powder to what's remaining and pulse to incorporate. Spread this chocolate layer over the prepared crust in a smooth layer. Transfer to the freezer to firm up, about 30 minutes.

ONCE the first layer is firm to the touch, evenly spread about one-half of the remaining vanilla filling on top of the chocolate layer and return the cheesecake to the freezer for 30 minutes.

RETURN what's left of the vanilla filling to the bowl or blender's canister (this time, rinse the bowl or canister first). Add the freeze-dried strawberries and blend to incorporate.

ONCE the vanilla layer is firm, spread the strawberry layer on top, smoothing it out. Tap the pan sharply on the counter a few times to release any air bubbles.

FREEZE the cheesecake for at least 3 hours, or until completely firm before adding the ganache.

FOR THE GANACHE: Put the chopped chocolate in a bowl. Warm the coconut milk in a saucepan until just simmering. (You can also warm the coconut milk in the microwave for 30 seconds.) Pour the warmed milk over the chopped chocolate, making sure the milk covers the chocolate. Let the mixture stand for 2 minutes to give the chocolate time to soften. Stir the ganache until smooth.

SPREAD the ganache over the cheesecake. Serve immediately or wrap well and refrigerate or freeze until ready to serve.

IF stored in the freezer, let the cheesecake thaw in the refrigerator for at least 1 hour before serving, or let it thaw at room temperature for 15 minutes. I recommend running your knife under hot water to warm it up and drying it before cutting the cheesecake with the still-hot knife.

STORE slices of cheesecake tightly wrapped in the refrigerator for 5 days, or in the freezer for up to 3 months.

Tip

If you have a kitchen scale, weigh the filling when you take it from the food processor or blender to get two-thirds. The finished filling weighs about 650g, so you'll want to transfer 435g to a separate bowl. Zero out a bowl on the scale and put 435g filling in the bowl. You'll have one-third (215g) left in the processor. This is how I do it when I want to be precise, although at times I simply eyeball it!

CHAPTER THREE

Pies, Tarts, and Crumbles

A FEW TIPS AND TRICKS FOR SUCCESS:

Pies, tarts, and crumbles are all great make-ahead desserts: For fruit pies, cobblers, and crumbles, cover and store them in the refrigerator until ready to bake to serve a freshly baked pie or crumble. For tarts, make them in their entirety and store in the refrigerator for up to a day or two before serving.

Fresh fruit is best for most of these recipes, so I would recommend using it if you can. For certain recipes, like the Mixed Berry Crisp and Nectarine-Blueberry Crisp, frozen fruit works fine, just thaw and drain it first.

Make sure to let all the pies, tarts, and crumbles cool completely before serving so that the fruit sets, which will give you the cleanest cuts.

Prep time: 45 minutes
Bake time: 50 minutes
Total time: 1 hour 35 minutes
Yield: 12 slices

FOR THE CRUST

1½ cups (144g) blanched almond flour

½ cup (57g) tapioca flour

3 tablespoons ground flax seed

1 tablespoon coconut sugar

¼ teaspoon kosher salt

6 tablespoons (75g) refined coconut oil, chilled

2 tablespoons cold water

FOR THE FILLING

¼ cup refined coconut oil

2 tablespoons tapioca flour

½ cup coconut sugar

2 tablespoons pure maple syrup

2 tablespoons fresh lemon juice

1 tablespoon pure vanilla extract

2 teaspoons ground cinnamon

¼ teaspoon ground ginger

¼ teaspoon grated nutmeg

¼ teaspoon allspice

2 pounds apples, such as Honeycrisp, Granny Smith, and Jonagold, peeled, cored, and sliced into ¼-inch slices

FOR THE CRUMBLE TOPPING

1 cup (96g) blanched almond flour

2 tablespoons coconut flour

APPLE CRUMBLE PIE

PALEO · GRAIN-FREE · VEGAN · GLUTEN-FREE · DAIRY-FREE

Apple crumble pie has long been one of my favorite desserts. When I was a kid, we used to get apple crumble pies from the local health food store that were made in Julian—a town about an hour away that is famous for their apples and apple pie. My sister and I would sit on the kitchen counter when we got home and pick the crumble off the top of the pie. This version has the same buttery crust and snackable crumble topping, but the crust is actually vegan and the crumble is made with almond flour and flaked coconut to keep it Paleo. It's perfect for serving at any holiday celebration that calls for pie—or anytime you're craving a little bit of apple crumble!

PREHEAT the oven to 425°F.

FOR THE CRUST: Combine the almond flour, tapioca flour, ground flax seed, coconut sugar, salt, and coconut oil in the bowl of a food processor fitted with the metal blade. Or if you prefer, combine the ingredients in a mixing bowl to work by hand. Pulse, or blend with a pastry blender, until the mixture has the texture of coarse meal. Add the water and pulse or stir until the dough comes together. If you're mixing in a bowl, you may want to use your hands to bring the dough together at the end.

ON a lightly floured work surface, roll out the dough between two sheets of parchment paper or on a silicone baking mat into a 12-inch round. Carefully fit the dough in a 9-inch pie dish (not a deep-dish pie plate). If the dough breaks, that's okay! Press it back into place with your fingertips. Repair any holes or cracks in the same way. Chill the pie shell in the freezer while preparing the filling.

FOR THE FILLING: Melt the coconut oil in a saucepan over medium-low heat. Whisk in the tapioca flour to form a paste and then whisk in the coconut sugar, maple syrup, lemon juice, vanilla, cinnamon, ginger, nutmeg, and allspice. Bring to a boil, simmer for 3 minutes, and remove from the heat.

CONTINUES

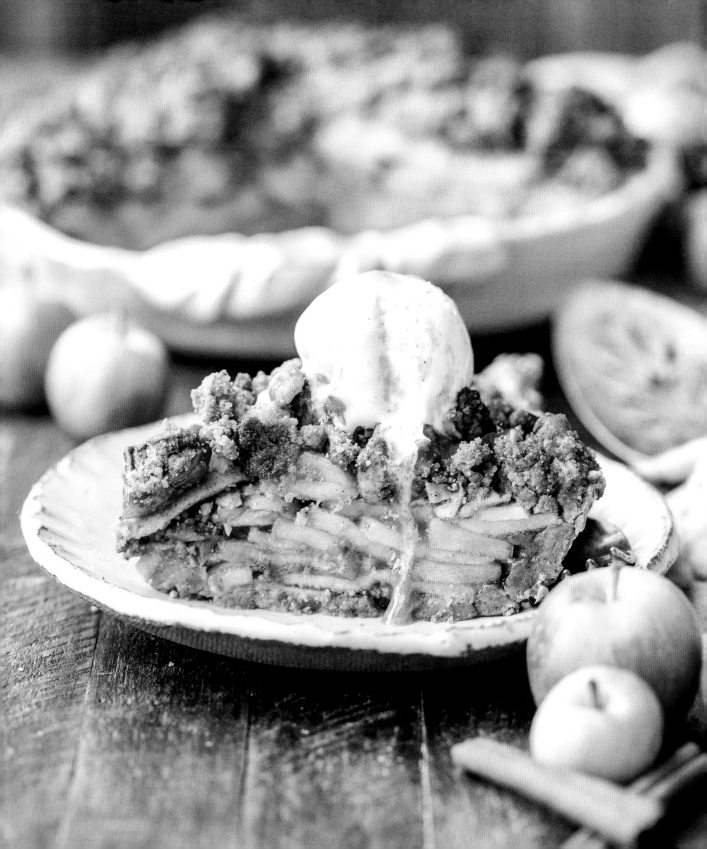

¼ cup (15g) flaked coconut, chopped into bits

¼ cup (85g) pure maple syrup

¼ cup (50g) refined coconut oil, softened

¼ cup (28g) chopped pecans

PUT the apples in a large bowl and pour the filling over them. Toss until the apples are coated. Pour the apples into the pie shell.

FOR THE CRUMBLE TOPPING: In a large mixing bowl, stir together the almond flour, coconut flour, flaked coconut, maple syrup, coconut oil, and pecans. Stir until the dry ingredients are completely moistened. Pick up the mixture with your fingers and crumble evenly over the apples.

PLACE the pie on a baking sheet and bake for 15 minutes. Reduce the temperature to 350°F and continue baking for 35 to 45 minutes longer, until the apples are tender and the crumble is golden brown on top. Tent with foil if the pie starts to brown too quickly!

LET the pie cool for at least 1 hour before serving. Serve warm or chilled. Keep any leftovers in the refrigerator for up to 4 days.

CHAI SPICE PEAR COBBLER

PALEO • GRAIN-FREE • VEGAN • GLUTEN-FREE • DAIRY-FREE

Pears are often under-loved in my kitchen, but this spiced pear cobbler reminded me that I love baking with pears so much! They're apples' juicier cousins and, in this cobbler, they melt into a delicious, buttery texture—not too firm, like apples can sometimes be, but also not too saucy. The combination of different pear varieties creates a mix of textures that delights the palate, and the warm flavors of the chai spices bring an unexpected flavor to the cobbler. Unlike a more traditional, biscuit-like cobbler, the topping here is similar to a fluffy batter going into the oven, which then puffs and browns for a cakey topping that is utterly delicious. Add a scoop of ice cream or some whipped coconut cream for a scrumptious dessert.

PREHEAT the oven to 375°F. Lightly grease an 8 × 8-inch pan or similarly sized round casserole dish with coconut oil.

FOR THE FILLING: In a bowl, toss the pear slices with the coconut sugar, tapioca flour, maple syrup, vanilla, cinnamon, nutmeg, ginger, cardamom, salt, and pepper until well mixed. Pour the fruit into the prepared pan.

FOR THE TOPPING: In a separate bowl, stir the almond flour with the tapioca flour, coconut oil, milk, coconut sugar, baking powder, vanilla, and salt. Mix until smooth and then dollop over the pears to cover.

FOR THE CINNAMON SUGAR: Stir together the coconut sugar and cinnamon and sprinkle over the batter.

BAKE the cobbler for 35 to 40 minutes, until a toothpick inserted into the topping comes out clean and the pears are bubbling.

Prep time: 20 minutes
Bake time: 35 minutes
Total time: about 1 hour
Yield: 8 servings

FOR THE FILLING
- 1½ pounds ripe firm fresh pears, such as Anjou and Bartlett, peeled, cored, and sliced into ¼-inch slices
- ⅓ cup coconut sugar
- 2 tablespoons plus 2 teaspoons tapioca flour
- 1 tablespoon pure maple syrup
- 1 teaspoon pure vanilla extract
- 1¼ teaspoons ground cinnamon
- ½ teaspoon grated nutmeg
- ½ teaspoon ground ginger
- ¼ teaspoon ground cardamom
- ¼ teaspoon kosher salt
- ⅛ teaspoon black pepper

FOR THE TOPPING
- ¾ cup (72g) blanched almond flour
- ¾ cup (85g) tapioca flour
- ⅓ cup (67g) coconut oil, melted
- ⅓ cup dairy-free milk, such as unsweetened almond milk
- 2 tablespoons coconut sugar
- 2¼ teaspoons baking powder
- 1 teaspoon pure vanilla extract
- Pinch of kosher salt

FOR THE CINNAMON SUGAR
- 2 teaspoons coconut sugar
- ¼ teaspoon ground cinnamon

Tip

Add 1 cup fresh cranberries to the pear mixture for some extra tartness and festive color!

Prep time: 15 minutes
Chill time: 2 hours
Total time: 2¼ hours
Yield: 10 slices

FOR THE HAZELNUT CRUST

1½ cups (168g) hazelnut meal
(see Tips)

¼ cup (50g) refined coconut oil,
melted

2 tablespoons pure maple syrup

¼ teaspoon kosher salt

FOR THE FILLING

6 ounces bittersweet chocolate,
finely chopped (I use
72 percent cacao)

¾ cup canned full-fat
coconut milk

⅓ cup Chocolate Hazelnut
Butter (page 269)

About 2 cups sliced fresh
strawberries (see Tips)

¼ cup chopped toasted
hazelnuts

- If you prefer more tartness,
substitute raspberries for
the strawberries, or you can
leave the berries out of the
recipe for an extra-rich and
decadent treat.
- Hazelnut meal can be
bought at the store, but you
can also make it yourself
by pulsing hazelnuts in a
blender or food processor
until fine and flour-like.

CHOCOLATE-HAZELNUT TART WITH STRAWBERRIES

PALEO • GRAIN-FREE • VEGAN • NO-BAKE • GLUTEN-FREE • DAIRY-FREE

For a long part of my life, I thought I didn't like hazelnuts. That was because I didn't like the ever-popular processed chocolate hazelnut spread, so I assumed I didn't like hazelnuts themselves. Once I tried a homemade version of chocolate hazelnut butter, I fell in love with the toasted, nutty flavor of the hazelnut, particularly when it's paired with chocolate—but nothing too milky or overly sweetened. This tart highlights the flavor of hazelnuts with a hazelnut meal crust and a chocolate filling that's made in part with homemade chocolate hazelnut butter. The decadent chocolate filling is topped off with fresh strawberries, which help cut through the richness of the chocolate, and chopped hazelnuts for a little crunch.

FOR THE CRUST: Lightly grease a 9-inch tart pan with a removable bottom with coconut oil.

IN a mixing bowl, stir together all the ingredients for the crust. When the dough comes together, press it evenly into the prepared tart pan, making sure to press it up the sides of the pan. Refrigerate to firm it up while you make the filling.

FOR THE FILLING: Put the finely chopped chocolate in a heat-proof mixing bowl. In a small saucepan, bring the coconut milk just to a boil. Pour the hot coconut milk over the chocolate and let the mixture stand for about 1 minute, then stir until smooth and creamy. Stir in the chocolate hazelnut butter until smooth. Pour the filling into the prepared crust in an even layer. Garnish the tart with strawberries and hazelnuts.

REFRIGERATE the tart for at least 2 hours to set and cool completely. Slice and serve. Refrigerate leftovers in an airtight container for up to 2 days.

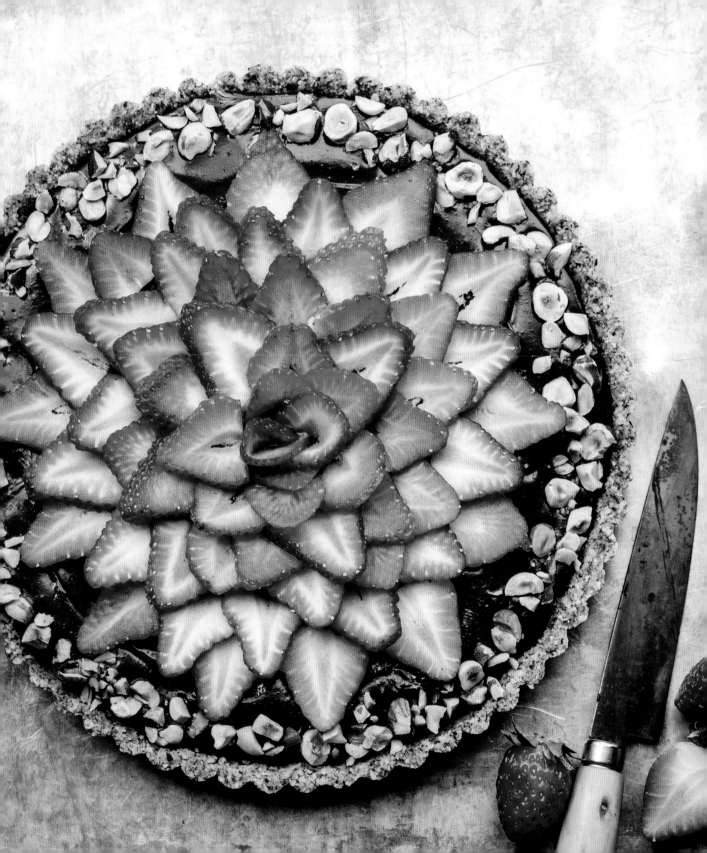

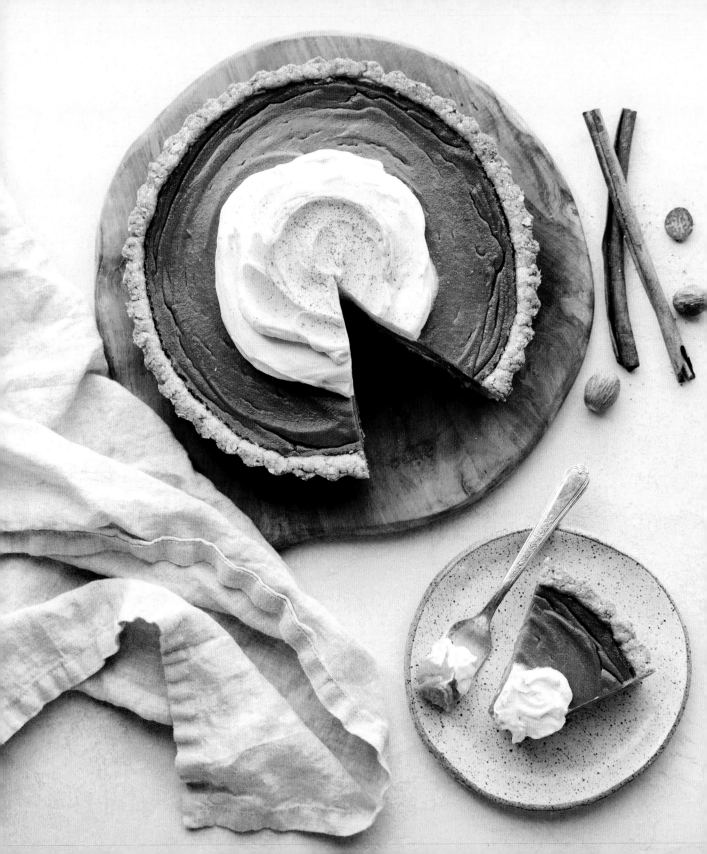

BUTTERNUT SQUASH PIE WITH OAT CRUST

VEGAN • GLUTEN-FREE • DAIRY-FREE

Move over, pumpkin pie—there's a new squash pie in town! Pumpkin has become standard on our holiday tables, but I find butternut squash to have a flavor that's even sweeter and more delicious than pumpkin. This pie uses roasted butternut squash in place of the more traditional canned pumpkin for a standout pie. The scents of maple syrup, cinnamon, nutmeg, ginger, and vanilla waft from the oven as the pie bakes in its oatmeal crust, and when it's served with a hearty scoop of whipped coconut cream on top, you'll want to devour every bite. This one is a new holiday staple for me!

BEFORE you begin, roast the squash for the filling. Preheat the oven to 350°F and line a baking sheet with parchment paper. Cut the squash in half lengthwise. Put the squash, cut-side down, on the baking sheet and roast for 45 to 60 minutes, until a knife easily pierces the squash through to the center. Let the squash cool slightly, remove the skin and seeds, and then measure 2½ cups of slightly mashed squash to use in the filling. Reserve any remaining squash for another use.

FOR THE CRUST: Keep the oven heated to 350°F (or heat it now, if you cooked the squash in advance). Thoroughly grease a 9-inch deep-dish pie plate or deep tart pan (at least 2 inches deep) with coconut oil.

IN a large mixing bowl, whisk the almond flour with the quick oats, baking powder, cinnamon, and salt until well mixed. Add the coconut oil and maple syrup and use a spoon to mix until all the dry ingredients are incorporated and no chunks of coconut oil remain.

PRESS the dough into the prepared pie pan, making sure to cover the bottom evenly and press the dough up the sides. (I like to use the base of a flat-bottomed measuring cup to press in the sides and make sure the bottom is flat.)

Prep time: 1 hour 15 minutes

Bake time: 45 minutes

Total time: 2 hours (plus 30 minutes cooling in the oven and 2 hours chilling)

Yield: 12 slices

1 butternut squash, about 1 pound

FOR THE CRUST

1½ cups (144g) blanched almond flour

1 cup (96g) gluten-free quick oats

1 teaspoon baking powder

1 teaspoon ground cinnamon

½ teaspoon kosher salt

⅓ cup (67g) refined coconut oil, softened (see Tip)

¼ cup (85g) pure maple syrup

FOR THE FILLING

¾ cup canned full-fat coconut milk

⅔ cup (96g) coconut sugar

¼ cup (28g) tapioca flour

2 tablespoons creamy almond butter

2 tablespoons pure maple syrup

1 tablespoon ground cinnamon

1 teaspoon ground ginger

1 teaspoon pure vanilla extract

¼ teaspoon ground nutmeg

¼ teaspoon allspice

¼ teaspoon kosher salt

⅛ teaspoon ground cloves

CONTINUES

FOR THE GARNISH
1 (13.5-ounce) can full-fat coconut cream, chilled overnight

Ground cinnamon, for dusting

Tip

The coconut oil should be the texture of softened butter. If it melts to a liquid because the kitchen is too warm, refrigerate for 15 to 20 minutes until it solidifies.

FOR THE FILLING: Combine the reserved 2½ cups of squash and the other filling ingredients in a blender or food processor fitted with the metal blade. Blend until completely smooth, scraping down the sides of the blender or food processor bowl as necessary. Pour the filling into the pie shell and tap against the counter a few times to release any air bubbles.

PLACE the pie on a baking sheet and bake for about 45 minutes, until the sides are set and the center jiggles only slightly when the pan is gently shaken.

TURN off the oven and prop the door open with a wooden spoon. Let the pie cool in the oven for 30 minutes. Transfer the pie to a wire rack to cool to room temperature, then cover with plastic wrap and refrigerate for at least 2 hours, or up to 12 hours before serving.

TO SERVE: Drain any liquid from the can of coconut cream. (Keep this liquid or not; it's good in smoothies.) Transfer the thick cream to a mixing bowl or the bowl of a stand mixer fitted with the whisk attachment. Whisk the chilled coconut cream by hand or in the mixer until creamy, about 30 seconds. Spread the coconut cream over the top of the pie. With a fine-mesh strainer, dust the coconut cream with cinnamon and serve immediately.

CHOCOLATE-PEANUT BUTTER TART

GRAIN-FREE • VEGAN • NO-BAKE • GLUTEN-FREE • DAIRY-FREE

It's a rare day that goes by that I don't have chocolate and peanut butter in one form or another. The obsession was likely sparked by my dad's love for the combo and his insistence on getting chocolate peanut butter cups whenever life called for candy. This tart is essentially one giant chocolate peanut butter cup—it has a chocolate crust filled with a lightly sweetened peanut butter filling, all topped off with a mixture of melted chocolate and peanut butter. A dusting of flaky sea salt on top balances out the sweetness and adds a little sophistication. Even better? No baking is required, so this is perfect to whip up on the days when you just don't feel like turning on the oven. Enjoy, my fellow chocolate peanut butter lovers!

FOR THE CRUST: Lightly grease a 9-inch tart pan with a removable bottom with coconut oil.

IN a mixing bowl, combine all the ingredients for the crust and stir together until everything is moistened. Press evenly into the bottom and up the sides of the prepared tart pan. Refrigerate while making the filling.

FOR THE FILLING: In a mixing bowl, stir together the peanut butter, maple syrup, coconut flour, and kosher salt if using, until smooth. Spread the filling into the prepared tart shell and use a spoon or offset spatula to spread it evenly. Refrigerate for about 30 minutes to set the filling.

FOR THE CHOCOLATE TOPPING: Once the filling is set, microwave the chocolate and peanut butter in a microwave-safe bowl for 30 seconds. Stir and then microwave in 15-second intervals, stirring between each, until the mixture is completely melted and smooth.

SPREAD the melted chocolate over the filling and garnish with chopped peanuts and flaky sea salt, as desired. Refrigerate for 1 hour to let the tart set before slicing and serving.

WRAP the tart in plastic wrap and store in an airtight container in the refrigerator for up to 1 week, or in the freezer for up to 2 months.

Prep time: 15 minutes
Chill time: 1 hour 30 minutes
Total time: 1¾ hours
Yield: 10 slices

FOR THE CRUST

1½ cups (144g) blanched almond flour

¼ cup (24g) cacao powder

¼ cup (50g) refined coconut oil, melted

2 tablespoons pure maple syrup

¼ teaspoon kosher salt

FOR THE FILLING

1½ cups (192g) creamy peanut butter

5 tablespoons (105g) pure maple syrup

⅓ cup (43g) coconut flour

¼ teaspoon kosher salt (skip if the nut butter is salted)

FOR THE CHOCOLATE TOPPING AND GARNISH

3 ounces bittersweet chocolate, chopped (about ½ cup)

2 tablespoons creamy peanut butter (see Tip)

Chopped roasted peanuts, for garnish

Flaky sea salt, for garnish

Tip

Although I love this with peanut butter, you can use another nut butter if you prefer.

Prep time: 15 minutes
Bake time: 30 minutes
Total time: 45 minutes
Yield: 9 servings

FOR THE BERRY FILLING
- **3 generous cups mixed berries, such as strawberries, raspberries, and blueberries (about 3 pints; see Tips)**
- **3 tablespoons pure maple syrup**
- **1 teaspoon pure vanilla extract**
- **2 tablespoons tapioca flour**

FOR THE ALMOND-BUTTER CRUMBLE TOPPING
- **2 tablespoons refined coconut oil, slightly softened (see Tips)**
- **⅓ cup (85g) creamy almond butter**
- **½ cup (64g) coconut flour**
- **½ cup (48g) gluten-free rolled oats**
- **¼ cup (28g) sliced almonds**
- **¼ cup (36g) coconut sugar**
- **1 teaspoon ground cinnamon**
- **¼ teaspoon kosher salt**

FOR THE GARNISH
- **1 (13.5-ounce) can full-fat coconut cream, chilled overnight**
- **¼ cup (64g) creamy almond butter**

MIXED BERRY CRISP WITH ALMOND-BUTTER CRUMBLE
VEGAN • GLUTEN-FREE • DAIRY-FREE

Fans of crumble toppings: Gather round, because this is one of the best crumbles I've had. Made with almond butter, the topping has a melt-in-your-mouth texture, and the rolled oats and sliced almonds add some bite. When piled on top of a mixture of fresh berries, it makes for a delectable dessert. You can also use thawed frozen berries here (see Tips), so you can make this all year round—no need to wait for summer berry season. Switch out the almond butter in the crumble for peanut butter and you'll have a version of PB&J that will make you drool!

PREHEAT the oven to 350°F. Lightly oil an 8×8-inch baking pan with coconut oil.

FOR THE FILLING: In a large mixing bowl, stir together the berries, maple syrup, vanilla, and tapioca flour until well mixed. Pour the filling into the prepared pan and gently spread it out to cover the bottom of the pan.

FOR THE TOPPING: In a separate bowl, mix together the coconut oil and almond butter until well blended. Add the coconut flour, oats, almonds, coconut sugar, cinnamon, and salt. Mix until the dry ingredients are incorporated and then crumble the mixture evenly over the berries.

BAKE the crisp for 30 minutes, until the berry filling is bubbling and the top is firm and lightly browned.

TO SERVE: Drain any liquid from the cans of coconut cream and transfer the thick cream to a mixing bowl or the bowl of a stand mixer fitted with the whisk attachment. Whisk the chilled coconut cream by hand or in the mixer for about 30 seconds or until creamy.

PUT the almond butter in a microwave-safe bowl and microwave for 15 seconds, or until thin and drizzly. Serve each piece of the crisp with a dollop of whipped coconut cream and a drizzle of almond butter.

- If you want, substitute frozen berries for the fresh berries. Thaw them slightly in a colander to release any excess water before using. Measure the berries after thawing.
- The coconut oil should be the consistency of softened butter. If it is supersoft or melted because the kitchen is too warm, refrigerate it for 15 to 30 minutes to firm it up.

Prep time: 15 minutes
Bake time: 40 minutes
Total time: about 1 hour
Servings: 8 to 10 slices

....

FOR THE FILLING

3 cups hulled and diced fresh strawberries (about 2 pints)

1 teaspoon fresh lemon juice

1 tablespoon pure maple syrup

1 tablespoon tapioca flour

FOR THE CRUST

1¼ cups (120g) blanched almond flour

¾ cup (72g) gluten-free rolled oats

1 teaspoon baking powder

¼ teaspoon kosher salt

Grated zest of 1 small lemon

¼ cup (85g) pure maple syrup

⅓ cup (67g) refined coconut oil, softened (see Tips)

¼ cup (28g) chopped pecans

STRAWBERRY CRUMBLE TART WITH OATMEAL CRUST

VEGAN • GLUTEN-FREE • DAIRY-FREE

When it's summer in San Diego, I'm always loaded up with pints upon pints of strawberries from the farmers' market. While strolling through my favorite Sunday market, the scent of sweet strawberries basking in the sun overtakes all the other competing scents and it's hard to not buy them all. Once I'm stuffed full of fresh, sun-kissed berries, I want to bake with them, and this crumble tart is perfect to highlight strawberries' fresh, sweet flavor. Tossed with just a bit of lemon juice, maple syrup, and tapioca starch, their flavor is allowed to shine, while being complemented by the lemon-scented oatmeal crust. It's healthy enough to eat for breakfast, but scrumptious enough for dessert—especially topped with some whipped coconut cream or vanilla ice cream.

....

PREHEAT the oven to 350°F; lightly grease a 9-inch tart pan with a removable bottom (see Tips) with coconut oil.

FOR THE FILLING: In a medium mixing bowl, toss together the strawberries, lemon juice, maple syrup, and tapioca flour until the berries are coated. Set the berries aside to macerate while you make the crust.

FOR THE CRUST: In a mixing bowl, whisk the almond flour with the oats, baking powder, salt, and zest until well mixed. Add the maple syrup and coconut oil and mix with a spoon or rubber spatula until the dough holds together when pressed between your fingers.

MEASURE a heaping ½ cup of the dough into a bowl. Add the chopped pecans and stir well. Set the crumble dough aside.

PUT the remaining dough in the prepared tart pan and press evenly into and up the sides of the pan. Pour the strawberries into the tart shell, making sure most of the juices remain in the bowl. Spread the berries evenly in the shell and sprinkle with the reserved crumble dough as evenly as you can.

CONTINUES

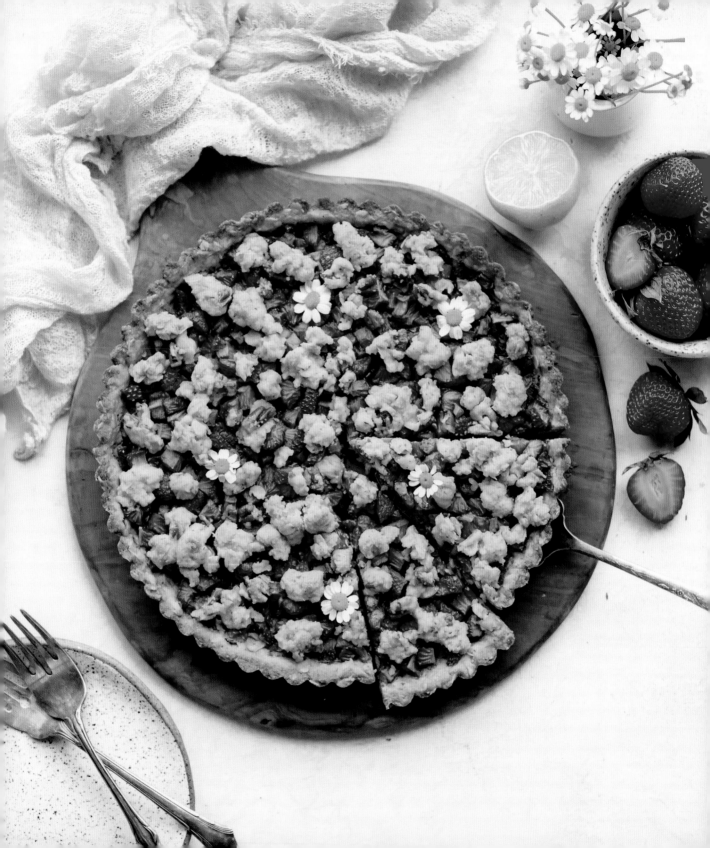

BAKE for about 40 minutes, until the filling is bubbling and the crust is golden brown. After 25 minutes of baking, tent the tart with foil to prevent it from getting too brown. Let the tart cool completely on a wire rack. When cool, slice the tart into 8 to 10 wedges and serve. Refrigerate the tart, well wrapped, for up to 1 week.

Tips

- The coconut oil should be the consistency of softened butter. If it is supersoft or melted because the kitchen is too warm, refrigerate it for 15 to 30 minutes to firm it up.
- This tart gets better with time and will be just as good on day two or three as it is on day one, thus making it a perfect make-ahead dessert.
- If you don't have a tart pan, the recipe works wonderfully as bar cookies. Bake in a lightly greased 8 × 8-inch pan and then slice into small square bars.

MANGO TART

PALEO • GRAIN-FREE • VEGAN • GLUTEN-FREE • DAIRY-FREE

There was an iconic mango tart at a local restaurant near where I grew up in Del Mar, California. While the tart had a crisp shortbread crust and a sweet vanilla filling, the real star was the always-perfectly-ripe mango slices that were crafted into a beautiful rose shape on top of the filling. The result was a tart that was naturally sweet and fruity, while satisfying all your dessert cravings . . . and was a feast for your eyes! My re-creation of the tart features a coconut-flavored crust that I think pairs beautifully with the ripe mangoes, and a whipped coconut cream filling for a creamy complement to the mangoes. Make sure your mangoes are ripe and bright orange—that makes for the most delicious version of this tart.

PREHEAT the oven to 350°F. Grease a 9-inch tart pan with a removable bottom with coconut oil.

FOR THE CRUST: In a mixing bowl, whisk the almond flour with the shredded coconut and salt. Add the coconut oil and maple syrup and mix until the mixture resembles coarse crumbs and clumps together when squeezed between your fingers.

TRANSFER the dough to the prepared tart pan and press it evenly over the bottom and up the sides of the pan. Use your fingers or the bottom of a flat-bottomed measuring cup.

BAKE the tart shell in the center of the oven until golden brown and firm, 12 to 14 minutes. Transfer to a wire rack to cool completely.

FOR THE FILLING: Drain the liquid from the chilled can of coconut cream. (Keep this liquid or not; it's good in smoothies.) Scoop the thick cream from the can and transfer it to a large bowl or the bowl of a stand mixer fitted with the whisk attachment. With a handheld whisk or the mixer, whip the coconut cream until fluffy. Add the maple syrup and vanilla and whisk again until combined. Refrigerate until you're ready to assemble the tart.

CONTINUES

Prep Time: 40 minutes
Bake Time: 12 minutes
Total Time: about 1 hour (plus cooling the tart crust)
Yield: 10 servings

FOR THE CRUST

- 1½ cups (144g) blanched almond flour
- ½ cup (57g) unsweetened finely shredded coconut
- ¼ teaspoon kosher salt
- 2 tablespoons virgin coconut oil, melted
- 2 tablespoons pure maple syrup

FOR THE FILLING

- 1 (13.5-ounce) can full-fat coconut cream, chilled overnight
- 2 tablespoons pure maple syrup
- 1 teaspoon pure vanilla extract
- 3 large or 5 small ripe mangoes

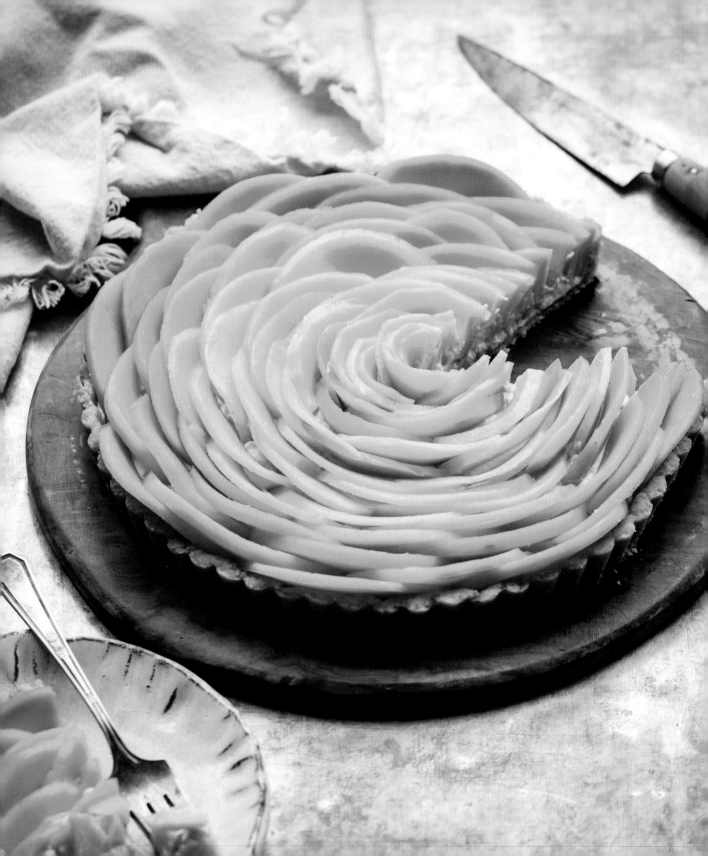

PEEL the mangoes with a vegetable peeler or small, sharp knife. Using your fingertips, balance the peeled mango upright on the counter. Position the knife to one side of the center stem and slice straight down, cutting as closely as possible to the large center pit. Turn the mango and slice off the other "cheek." You will have 2 large pieces of mango and the flat pit. Discard the pit. Slice the mango cheeks lengthwise into very thin strips. Repeat with the other mangoes.

SPREAD the chilled whipped coconut cream in an even layer over the completely cooled crust.

STARTING with the longest strips of mango, arrange the slices around the edge of the tart. Repeat, working your way toward the center, slightly overlapping the rows. When you reach the center of the tart, roll a mango slice into a curl and put it in the center. Serve right away or keep the tart covered and refrigerated until serving. It's best the day it's made but will keep, covered, for up to 3 days in the refrigerator.

Prep time: 15 minutes
Bake time: 50 minutes
Total time: about 1 hour
Yield: 8 servings

FOR THE FILLING
3 fresh nectarines (about 1 pound), peeled, pitted, and chopped into ½-inch pieces

1½ cups fresh blueberries (about 1¾ pints)

2 tablespoons coconut sugar

2 tablespoons tapioca flour

1 teaspoon grated lemon zest

1 tablespoon fresh lemon juice

½ teaspoon ground cinnamon

FOR THE CRUMBLE
1 cup (96g) blanched almond flour

⅓ cup (57g) cornmeal

¼ cup (36g) coconut sugar

¼ teaspoon kosher salt

1 tablespoon pure maple syrup

¼ cup (50g) refined coconut oil, softened (see Tips)

NECTARINE-BLUEBERRY CRISP WITH CORNMEAL CRUMBLE
VEGAN • GLUTEN-FREE • DAIRY-FREE

When stone fruits pile up at the farmers' market for the first time in late summer, I end up with bags of ripe nectarines at my house. Most get devoured by themselves—their ripe, sweet flavor is enough all on its own. But inevitably, I want to bake some of them into a bubbly, sweet crisp. Paired with blueberries in this one, the two fruits are lightly sweetened with maple, scented with lemon, and topped with a cornmeal crumble. The cornmeal adds a delicious and unique flavor and texture to the topping, which pairs so well with the fruits. Serve with ice cream for dessert, or with coconut yogurt for breakfast!

PREHEAT the oven to 350°F. Lightly grease an 8 × 8-inch pan or similarly sized round casserole dish with coconut oil.

FOR THE FILLING: In a large bowl, mix the nectarine pieces with the blueberries. Add the coconut sugar, tapioca flour, lemon zest and juice, and cinnamon and toss to coat the fruit. Pour into the prepared pan and spread the fruit evenly.

FOR THE CRUMBLE: In the same or another mixing bowl, toss the almond flour with the cornmeal, coconut sugar, and salt. Stir in the maple syrup and coconut oil until the mixture comes together in a crumbly dough.

PRESS the dough into clumps and crumble them over the top of the fruit mixture. (You might have more crumble than you need, depending on the size of the pan and how much topping you like. If so, use it for another crumble.)

BAKE the crisp for 50 to 60 minutes, until the top is golden brown and the fruit is bubbling. If the crisp is browning more than you like, cover it with aluminum foil to prevent it from browning further.

LET the crisp cool for at least 10 minutes before serving.

Tips

- If you prepare this ahead of time to bake later, cover it with plastic wrap after adding the crumble. Refrigerate for up to 24 hours.
- The coconut oil should be the consistency of softened butter. If it is supersoft or melted because the kitchen is too warm, refrigerate it for 15 to 30 minutes to firm it up.

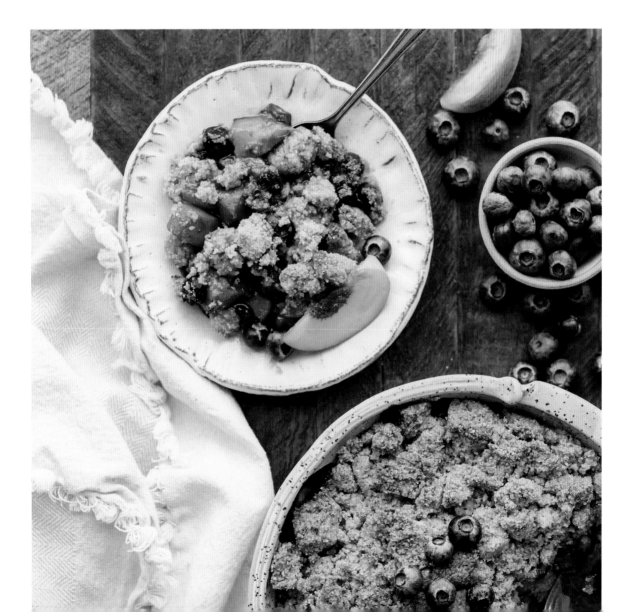

Prep time: 25 minutes
Chill time: 2 hours
Total time: About 2½ hours
Yield: 10 slices

1 small (10-ounce) sweet potato

FOR THE CRUST
¾ cup (72g) blanched almond
    flour

1¼ cups (141g) raw pecans

3 tablespoons coconut sugar

3 tablespoons refined coconut
    oil, melted

½ teaspoon ground cinnamon

¼ teaspoon kosher salt

FOR THE FILLING
⅔ cup canned full-fat coconut
    milk

⅓ cup cacao powder

¼ cup pure maple syrup

3 tablespoons cacao butter,
    melted

1 tablespoon pure vanilla extract

½ teaspoon kosher salt

FOR THE GARNISH
1 (13.5-ounce) can full-fat
    coconut cream, chilled
    overnight

¼ cup pomegranate seeds

CHOCOLATE MOUSSE PIE
PALEO • GRAIN-FREE • VEGAN • NO-BAKE • GLUTEN-FREE • DAIRY-FREE

You might look at the first ingredient in this pie and get skeptical.
Just trust me on this one—this chocolate mousse pie is a great party
trick. I had a grand old time letting people guess what was in the
pie, and then watching all of their faces turn to shock when they
learned the base of the creamy chocolate filling is the humble sweet
potato. Yes: An entire sweet potato serves as the main ingredient in
the filling, and, while it adds a smooth, creamy texture and a bit of
sweetness, you'd never guess it was there unless you made it yourself.

BEFORE you begin, cook the sweet potato for the filling. Pierce
the sweet potato in several places with a fork and then wrap
it in a damp paper towel. Put it on a microwave-safe plate and
microwave for 3 minutes. Turn the sweet potato over, leaving the
paper towel in place. Microwave for another 3 minutes, or until
the potato is tender and cooked all the way through. Depending
on the shape of the potato, it might take a little more or less time
to cook through. Alternatively, you can bake the sweet potato at
350°F for 45 minutes, until tender. Let the sweet potato cool for
5 to 10 minutes and then remove the skin. Set it aside to use later
while you make the crust.

FOR THE CRUST: Lightly grease a 6-inch springform pan or an
8-inch tart pan with a removable bottom with coconut oil.

COMBINE the almond flour, pecans, coconut sugar, coconut oil,
ground cinnamon, and salt in the bowl of a food processor fitted
with the metal blade or high-powered blender (I use a Vitamix). Pulse
until the pecans are broken up and the dough is fully moistened
and sticks together. Scrape down the sides of the bowl or blender as
necessary.

PRESS the dough evenly along the bottom and up the sides of the
prepared pan.

CONTINUES

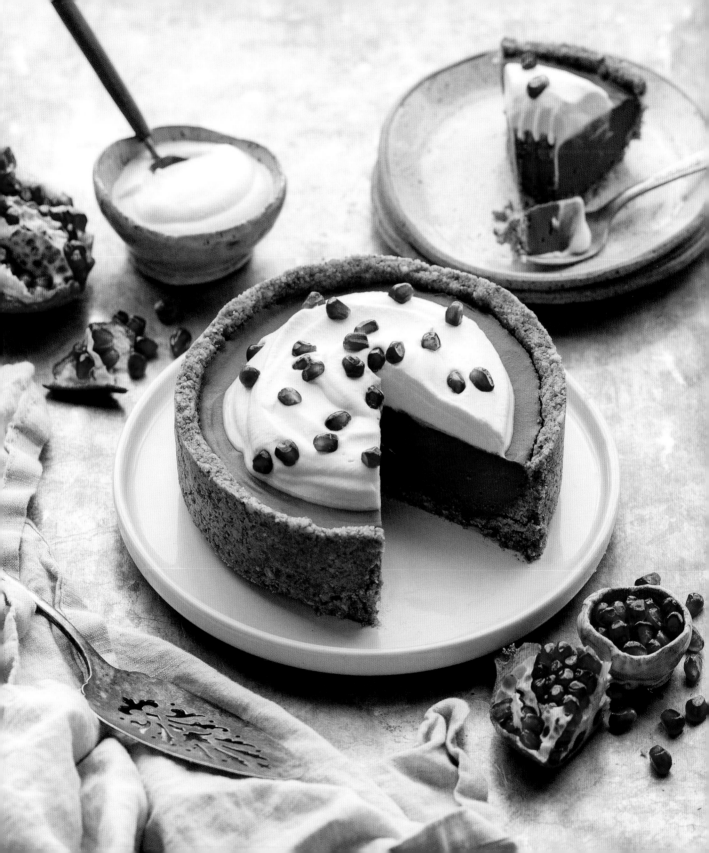

FOR THE FILLING: In a blender or bowl of a food processor fitted with the metal blade, combine the cooked sweet potato, coconut milk, cacao powder, maple syrup, melted cacao butter, vanilla, and salt. Blend or pulse on medium speed until completely smooth, scraping down the sides of the canister or bowl as necessary, about 2 minutes. If using a blender, use the tamper to keep things moving.

POUR the filling into the prepared pie shell and smooth the top. Refrigerate for at least 2 hours to firm up.

TO SERVE: Drain the liquid from the can of coconut cream. (Keep this liquid or not; it's good in smoothies.) Transfer the cream to a bowl and whisk until smooth and fluffy, about 30 seconds. Garnish the pie with the whipped coconut cream or pomegranate seeds, or both. Refrigerate well covered for up to 5 days.

SALTED MAPLE PECAN TART WITH PRETZEL SHORTBREAD CRUST

VEGAN · GLUTEN-FREE · DAIRY-FREE

I'm a sucker for anything with a big dusting of flaky sea salt on top. You might've noticed that I have a penchant for sprinkling it on anything with chocolate or caramel—it adds an irresistible counter to the sweetness of desserts and brings out the more savory flavors that are sometimes overshadowed. In this tart, we have salt two ways: coating the pretzels that are crushed into the shortbread crust, and in the form of flaky sea salt that's sprinkled generously over the top of the tart, finding its way between the pecan crevices to get into every bite. The salt blends magically with the flavor of the maple syrup, taming its sweetness. With a scoop of whipped coconut cream on top, you have a dessert elegant enough to serve at a dinner party and so delicious you'll want to sneak a slice from the fridge long after the party is over!

PREHEAT the oven to 350°F. Grease a 9-inch tart pan with a removable bottom with coconut oil.

FOR THE CRUST: In a blender, pulse the pretzels until no big chunks remain but they are not yet powdery.

IN a large mixing bowl, mix together the coconut oil and maple syrup until fully combined. Stir in the crushed pretzels, coconut flour, and salt and mix until the dough is as smooth as possible. Press the dough into the prepared pan, making sure to press it up the sides. A flat-bottomed measuring cup helps with this.

BAKE for about 6 minutes, until the crust firms up but is not browned. Let the crust cool completely on a wire rack while you prepare the filling.

FOR THE FILLING: Whisk together the coconut sugar, maple syrup, and coconut oil in a small saucepan. Cook over medium-low heat, whisking constantly to prevent burning, until the mixture

Prep time: 30 minutes
Bake time: 30 minutes
Total time: 1 hour
Yield: 10 slices

FOR THE CRUST
⅓ cup (25g) gluten-free pretzels
⅓ cup (67g) refined coconut oil, melted
¼ cup (85g) pure maple syrup
1 cup (128g) coconut flour
¼ teaspoon kosher salt

FOR THE FILLING
½ cup (120g) coconut sugar
¼ cup (85g) pure maple syrup
¼ cup (50g) refined coconut oil, melted
⅓ cup dairy-free milk, such as unsweetened almond or coconut milk
2 tablespoons ground flax seed
2 teaspoons tapioca flour
1 teaspoon pure vanilla extract
½ teaspoon kosher salt
1¼ cups roughly chopped pecans
1 teaspoon flaky sea salt

CONTINUES

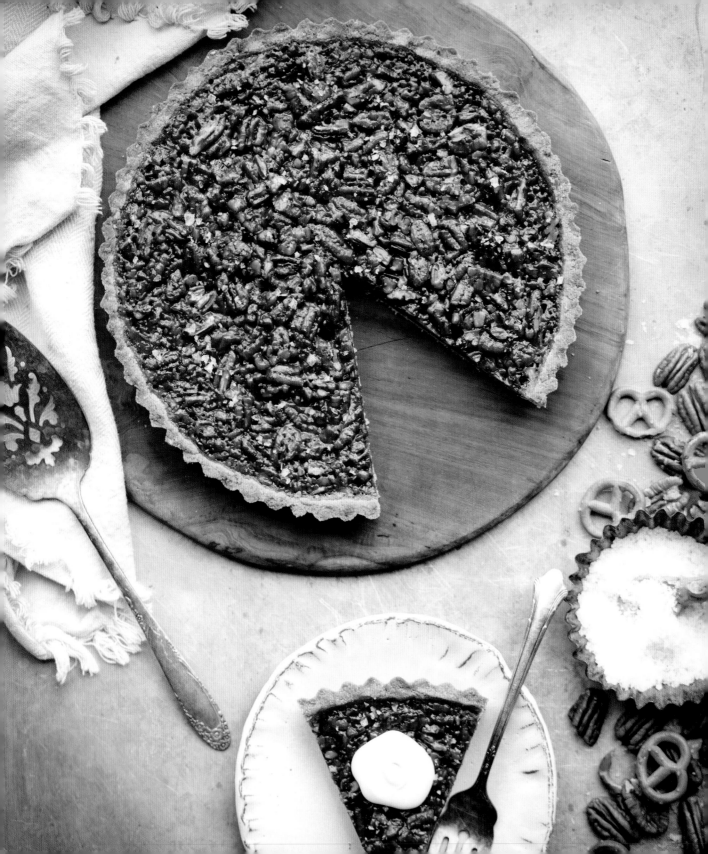

begins to boil. Adjust the heat and let the filling simmer for 2 to 3 minutes. Remove the pan from the heat and let cool slightly.

MEANWHILE, whisk together the milk, ground flax seed, tapioca flour, vanilla, and kosher salt in a small bowl.

ADD the milk mixture to the slightly cooled sugar mixture and whisk to combine. Stir in the pecans. Pour the filling over the cooled crust, spreading it as evenly as possible.

PLACE the tart on a baking sheet and bake for about 25 minutes, until the filling is hot and bubbling. Check after 15 minutes and if the crust is brown enough, tent it with foil to prevent further browning.

LET the tart cool completely on a wire rack, at least 2 hours. Sprinkle with the flaky sea salt and serve. Store in an airtight container in the refrigerator for up to 5 days.

CHAPTER FOUR

Cookies

A FEW TIPS AND TRICKS FOR SUCCESS:

To keep a constant supply of cookies on hand for when I need them, I'll make a batch of dough, form it into balls, place them on a parchment-covered plate or small baking sheet, and freeze the dough balls for a few hours, or until firm. Once they're hard, I throw them into a zippered bag and mark the bag with what's inside, the date when they were made, and the temperature and time to bake them. Then, when the cookie craving hits, all I've got to do is bake, adding about 2 minutes to the baking time. This can be done with all the drop cookies in this chapter, and they will keep in the freezer for about 6 months.

Cookie scoops are the best for making sure your cookies are all the same size! For all the drop cookies in this book, I use the medium cookie scoop from OXO, which holds 1½ tablespoons of dough and yields a cookie that's 2½ to 3 inches across. You can use a bigger or smaller scoop if preferred, but you'll need to adjust the baking time accordingly.

Cookie dough is pretty much always better after a chill in the refrigerator. It allows the flavors to meld and helps the cookies bake up thicker. If time allows, give your cookie dough at least 1 hour (or up to 48 hours) to chill before baking.

Use parchment paper or a silicone baking mat to line the baking sheet. This helps prevent the cookies from spreading too much.

Though it may be tempting to bake all your cookies at once, it's best to bake only one sheet in the oven at a time, on the center rack.

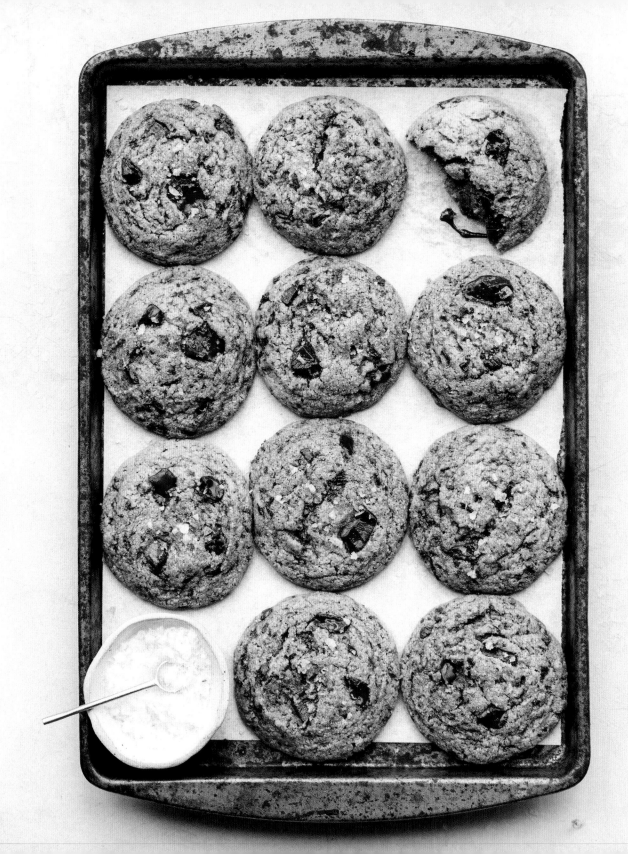

PALEO CHOCOLATE CHIP COOKIES

PALEO • GRAIN-FREE • VEGAN • GLUTEN-FREE • DAIRY-FREE

Anyone who asks me, "Which recipe from your blog should I try first?" gets the same response: Paleo chocolate chip cookies. When I asked my Instagram community which recipes from my site they'd like to see in my cookbook, this recipe was by far the most mentioned. It is also one of the few recipes that I make over and over and over again, no matter how many other treats I have in the house (even, um, if it's just to eat the dough). I simply can't resist the crisp, buttery edges and the doughy center filled with melted shards of chopped chocolate. These cookies can be made vegan by using a flax egg (also perfect for dough eating!) and is the perfect thing to feed to anyone who is convinced that they "don't like gluten-free desserts."

IN a mixing bowl or the bowl of a stand mixer fitted with the paddle attachment, beat the coconut sugar and coconut oil until smooth. Add the egg and vanilla and mix until smooth.

ADD the almond flour, baking soda, and salt to the wet ingredients. Mix until well incorporated. Fold in the chopped chocolate. Cover the bowl with plastic wrap and refrigerate for at least 1 hour or up to 48 hours, to give the flavors time to settle. (You can skip chilling the dough if you are short on time.)

PREHEAT the oven to 350°F; line a baking sheet with parchment paper.

USE a cookie scoop or spoon to form rounded cookies. Put them on the baking sheet and press to flatten slightly. Sprinkle with flaky sea salt, if desired. Bake for 10 to 12 minutes, until the cookies begin to turn golden brown around the edges. The exact time will depend on the size of the cookies.

STORE the baked cookies in an airtight container at room temperature for up to 5 days.

Prep time: 10 minutes

Bake time: 10 minutes

Total time: 20 minutes (plus optional 1 hour chilling)

Yield: 12 to 20 cookies, depending on size

⅔ cup (96g) coconut sugar

½ cup (100g) refined coconut oil, at room temperature

1 flax egg (see Tip) or 1 large egg, at room temperature

1 teaspoon pure vanilla extract

2¼ cups (216g) blanched almond flour

½ teaspoon baking soda

½ teaspoon kosher salt

6 ounces bittersweet chocolate, chopped (about 1 cup)

Flaky sea salt to sprinkle on top (optional)

Tip

To make a flax egg, mix 1 tablespoon ground flax seed with 2½ tablespoons water. Whisk well and then set aside at room temperature for about 10 minutes to gel.

Prep time: 15 minutes
Chill time: 1 hour
Bake time: 12 minutes
Total time: about 1½ hours
Yield: 15 cookies

FOR THE RASPBERRY CHIA JAM

1 cup fresh or frozen raspberries

1 tablespoon chia seeds

FOR THE COOKIES

1½ cups (144g) blanched almond flour

¼ cup (50g) refined coconut oil, melted

¼ cup (85g) pure maple syrup

¼ teaspoon kosher salt

Heaping ¼ cup shelled pistachios

Tip

It's tricky to make a smaller amount of jam than you need here. One batch will make enough for two batches of cookies, so you'll have some jam left over to use as you please.

PISTACHIO THUMBPRINT COOKIES WITH RASPBERRY JAM

PALEO • GRAIN-FREE • VEGAN • GLUTEN-FREE • DAIRY-FREE

For so many of us, baking conjures a sense of nostalgia. Whether it brings back memories of baking from scratch with your parents or grandparents (like me baking with my mom as a little girl) or makes you remember the simpler days where you were breaking out a roll of slice-and-bake cookies, it tends to be an activity that brings some flurry of emotion to mind. I think a lot of us probably remember making thumbprint cookies at some point in our childhood—I recall always making them in summer camp cooking classes. They're generally simple, hands-on, and absolutely delicious. This version, with pistachios and raspberry jam, are certainly all that. The pistachios add a wonderful crunch to the shortbread-like cookies and the tart raspberry jam brightens everything up. Maybe these will be the thumbprint cookies that your kids remember fondly when they're baking decades from now!

FOR THE RASPBERRY CHIA JAM: In a medium saucepan, lightly mash the raspberries and bring them to a simmer over medium heat, stirring frequently. After about 5 minutes the berries will start to break down. Add the chia seeds, stir to mix, and reduce the heat to medium-low. Continue cooking, uncovered and stirring frequently to prevent the bottom from burning until it cooks down a little, about 5 minutes. Remove from the heat; the jam will continue to thicken as it cools.

WHEN lukewarm or a little cooler, transfer the jam to a small jar or bowl and refrigerate to cool completely while you prepare the cookie dough.

FOR THE COOKIES: In a mixing bowl, stir together the almond flour, coconut oil, maple syrup, and salt until completely mixed and a thick dough forms. Form the dough into a ball, wrap with plastic wrap, and refrigerate for at least 1 hour to let the dough firm up, or up to 24 hours.

CONTINUES

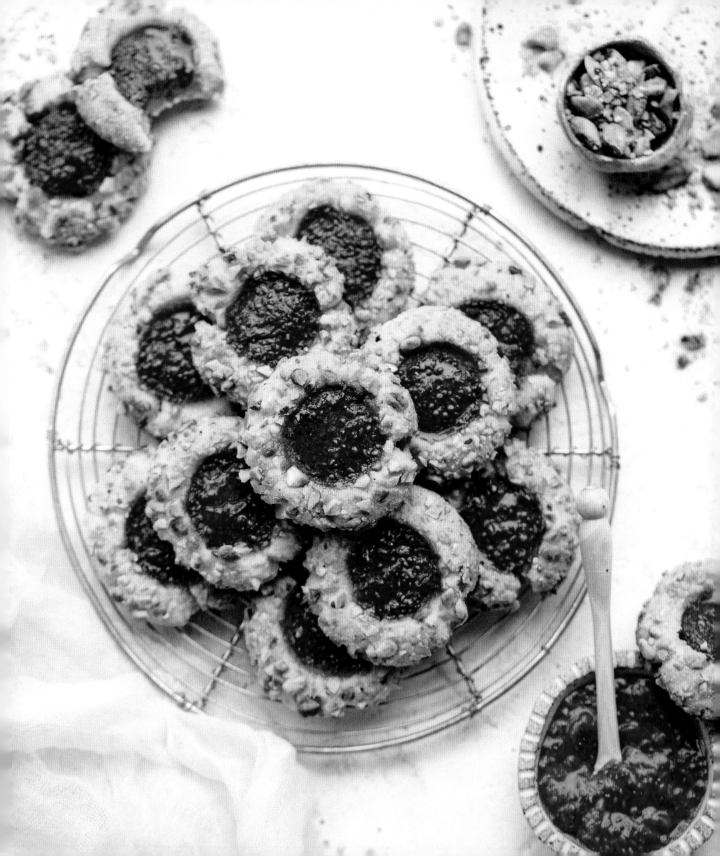

WHEN you're ready to bake, preheat the oven to 375°F; line a baking sheet with parchment paper.

PUT the pistachios in the bowl of a food processor fitted with the metal blade or a high-powered blender. Pulse until the nuts are in small bits. You will have about ¼ cup of nut pieces. Spread them on a work surface or plate.

FORM the chilled dough into 15 balls of dough, about 1 generous tablespoon each. Roll each ball in the ground pistachios and arrange on the baking sheet, leaving about 2 inches between each because they spread. Make an imprint in the center of each cookie with your thumb or a small, blunt tool (I use a cocktail muddler with a round, blunt end). Fill each imprint with about a teaspoon of the raspberry chia jam.

BAKE for 12 to 14 minutes, until the cookies are light golden brown around the edges. Let the cookies cool for 5 minutes on the baking sheet before transferring them to a wire rack to cool completely. Store in a covered container at room temperature for up to 5 days.

WHITE CHOCOLATE–MACADAMIA NUT COOKIES

PALEO • GRAIN-FREE • VEGAN • GLUTEN-FREE • DAIRY-FREE

White chocolate macadamia nut cookies have forever been one of my favorite cookies, right up there with chocolate chip cookies. The rich, buttery macadamia nuts paired with the luscious sweetness of white chocolate, all tucked into a sweet cookie dough—pure heaven for a cookie lover like me. But after going dairy-free, white chocolate was an issue. In the journey of recipe testing, as soon as I nailed a homemade white chocolate recipe (page 230) that would bake well, white chocolate macadamia nut cookies were a MUST-MAKE. These cookies are soft, rich, and sure to satisfy your craving.

IN a mixing bowl or the bowl of a stand mixer fitted with the paddle attachment, beat together the coconut oil and coconut sugar until smooth. Add the egg and vanilla and mix until smooth.

ADD the almond flour, salt, and baking soda to the wet ingredients. Mix until well incorporated. Fold in the chopped white chocolate and macadamia nuts. Cover with plastic wrap and refrigerate for at least 1 hour, or up to 48 hours.

WHEN you're ready to bake, preheat the oven to 350°F; line a baking sheet with parchment paper.

USE a cookie scoop to form cookies. Arrange on the baking sheet and gently press each to flatten a little. Bake for 10 to 12 minutes, until the cookies are just beginning to turn golden brown around the edges.

LET the cookies cool on the baking sheet for 10 minutes before transferring to a wire rack to cool completely.

STORE in an airtight container at room temperature for up to 5 days.

CONTINUES

Prep time: 10 minutes

Chill time: 1 hour

Bake time: 10 minutes

Total time: 1 hour 20 minutes

Yield: 15 to 20 cookies, depending on size

- ½ cup (100g) refined coconut oil, at room temperature
- ⅔ cup (96g) coconut sugar
- 1 flax egg (see Tips) or 1 large egg, at room temperature
- 1 teaspoon pure vanilla extract
- 2 cups plus 2 tablespoons (204g) blanched almond flour
- ½ teaspoon kosher salt
- ½ teaspoon baking soda
- 3 ounces dairy-free white chocolate (see Tips), chopped into chunks
- ½ cup chopped toasted macadamia nuts

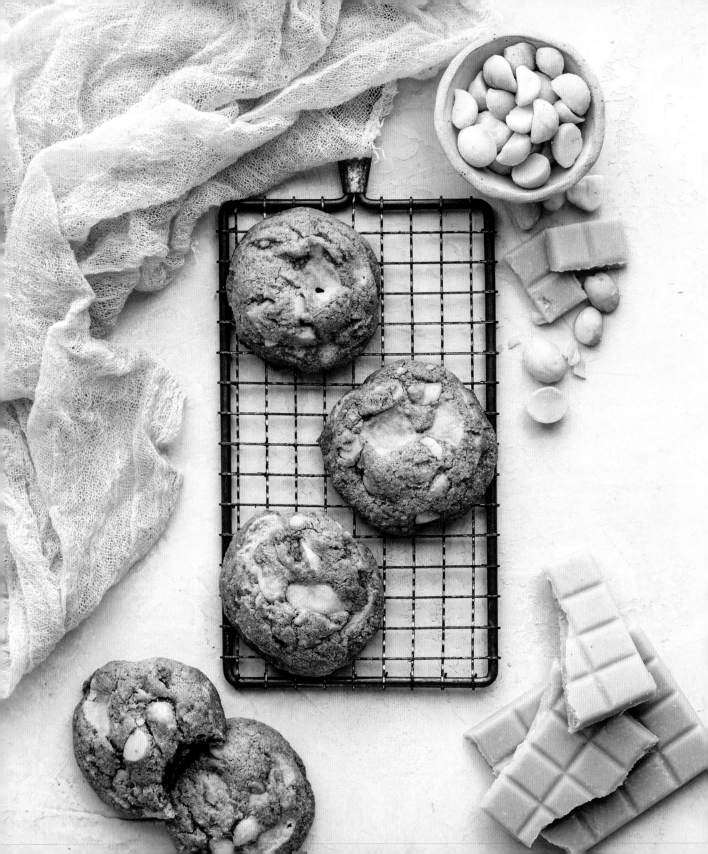

- I use my Homemade White Chocolate (page 230) for these cookies, but you can also use a ready-made dairy-free white chocolate, which can be found online or sometimes in the kosher section of the supermarket. Commercial white chocolate can be supersweet, so I suggest tasting beforehand. If you find it too sweet, I recommend reducing the amount of coconut sugar to ½ cup.
- To make a flax egg, whisk 1 tablespoon ground flax seed with 2½ tablespoons water. Set aside for about 10 minutes to give the mixture time to gel.

Prep time: 20 minutes

Chill time: 30 minutes

Bake time: 20 minutes

Total time: about 1¼ hours

Yield: about 20 cookies

FOR THE COOKIES

1 cup (96g) blanched almond flour

¼ cup (32g) arrowroot starch

⅛ teaspoon sea salt

3 tablespoons (63g) pure maple syrup

2 tablespoons refined coconut oil or ghee (see Tips), melted

½ teaspoon pure vanilla extract

½ cup (56g) very finely chopped pecans

FOR THE CHOCOLATE DIP

3 ounces bittersweet chocolate, chopped or as chips (about 6 tablespoons)

2 teaspoons refined coconut oil or cacao butter (see Tips)

Flaky sea salt, for sprinkling (optional)

CHOCOLATE-DIPPED PECAN CRESCENT COOKIES

PALEO • GRAIN-FREE • VEGAN • GLUTEN-FREE • DAIRY-FREE

As I taught myself to bake during childhood, I poured over cookbooks, meticulously baking different desserts. One favorite was a version of crescent cookies from a well-worn cookbook in my mom's kitchen—I adored the cookie's buttery texture and whimsical shape. The particular version that I made had pecans stirred into the stiff, buttery dough and were drizzled with milk chocolate. These chocolate-dipped pecan crescent cookies are my modern-day re-creation of those cookies—chock-full of pecan bits and dunked in chocolate (dark, this time around). If you're not strictly dairy-free or vegan, try using ghee in place of the coconut oil. It adds a scrumptious buttery flavor that will make your mouth water. The cookies are also perfect for gifting around the holidays—if you're willing to part with them, that is!

LINE a baking sheet with parchment paper.

FOR THE COOKIES: In a mixing bowl or bowl of a stand mixer fitted with the paddle attachment, mix the almond flour with the arrowroot starch and salt. Add the maple syrup, coconut oil, and vanilla extract and stir until combined. Fold in ¼ cup of the finely chopped pecans.

SHAPE about 2 teaspoons of dough into a crescent moon shape about ¼ inch thick and lay on the prepared baking sheet. Repeat with the remaining dough to make about 20 crescent-shaped cookies. If you want to flatten or even them out a bit, lightly roll over the tops with a rolling pin (or wine bottle). Refrigerate the cookies for at least 30 minutes, or up to 24 hours.

WHEN you're ready to bake, preheat the oven to 325°F.

PRESS the remaining ¼ cup chopped pecans into the cookie tops. I do this by putting the pecans on a plate and pressing half of the top of each cookie into the pecans.

CONTINUES

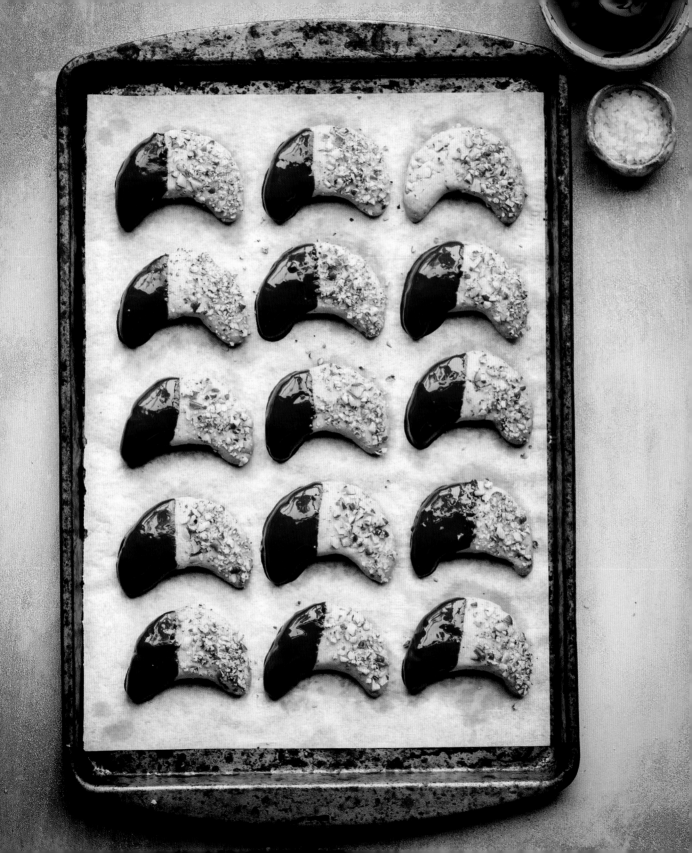

BAKE for 20 to 24 minutes, until golden brown around the edges. The longer they bake, the crispier the cookies will be, so watch them closely. Remove the cookies from the oven and let them cool completely on the baking sheet.

FOR THE CHOCOLATE DIP: Once the cookies are fully cooled, melt the chocolate and coconut oil together in a small microwave-safe bowl. Microwave for 1 minute and then stir. If the mixture is not fully melted, heat for another 30 seconds and stir again. You may have to microwave the mixture a third time.

DIP the half of each cookie without the pecans in the chocolate. Let the excess chocolate drip off and then return the cookies to the parchment-lined baking sheet. Repeat until all the cookies are coated. Sprinkle with flaky sea salt, if desired.

REFRIGERATE the cookies for at least 10 minutes to firm up the chocolate, and then serve. Store in an airtight container in the refrigerator for up to 1 week, or in the freezer for up to 3 months.

Tips

- For entirely dairy-free and vegan cookies, use coconut oil, not ghee.
- I recommend using cacao butter for the chocolate dip if you have it on hand. Because it has a higher melting point than coconut oil, it will stay firmer at room temperature and maintain a snappier texture.

NUT-FREE CHOCOLATE CHIP COOKIES

PALEO • GRAIN-FREE • NUT-FREE • VEGAN • GLUTEN-FREE • DAIRY-FREE

These chocolate chip cookies are so rich and decadent, with big chocolate chunks and a chewy texture—and they're also super allergen-friendly! They were developed out of a request for almond flour–free chocolate chip cookies, so this recipe uses coconut flour instead. Many coconut flour treats can end up dry and crumbly because it is such an absorbent flour (about three times more absorbent than other flours!), but since this recipe uses only ⅓ cup, the cookies stay rich, chewy, and not at all crumbly. They're kept vegan with flax eggs and can be made entirely nut-free by using tahini or sunflower seed butter. If you're not sensitive to nuts, any other nut butter can be used instead.

PREHEAT the oven to 350°F; line a baking sheet with parchment paper.

IN a bowl or stand mixer fitted with the paddle attachment, beat together the coconut oil, sunflower seed butter, and coconut sugar until smooth. Add the flax eggs and vanilla and mix until smooth.

ADD the coconut flour, baking soda, and salt to the wet ingredients. Mix until well incorporated. Fold in the chopped chocolate.

USE a cookie scoop to form cookies, then place 2 inches apart on the baking sheet. Sprinkle them with a little flaky sea salt, if desired. Bake for about 10 minutes, until the cookies are just beginning to turn golden brown around the edges.

COOL for 5 minutes on the baking sheet and then move to a wire rack to cool completely. Store in an airtight container at room temperature for up to 5 days.

CONTINUES

Prep time: 10 minutes
Bake time: 10 minutes
Total time: 20 minutes
Yield: 10 cookies

- ½ cup (100g) refined coconut oil, softened (see Tips)
- ⅓ cup (85g) sunflower seed butter or tahini (see Tips)
- ⅔ cup (96g) coconut sugar
- 2 flax eggs (see Tips)
- 1 teaspoon pure vanilla extract
- ⅓ cup (43g) coconut flour
- ½ teaspoon baking soda (if using sunflower seed butter, reduce the amount of baking soda to ¼ teaspoon to prevent the cookies from turning green when they cool!)
- ½ teaspoon kosher salt
- 4 ounces bittersweet chocolate, chopped (about ⅔ cup)
- Flaky sea salt, for sprinkling (optional)

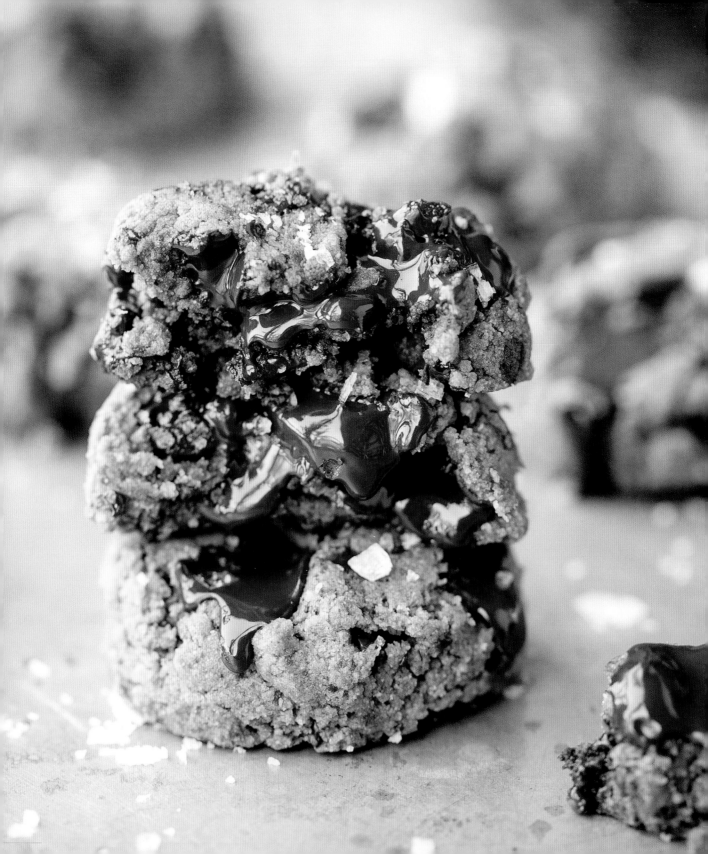

Tips

- The coconut oil should be the consistency of softened butter. If it gets too soft because the kitchen is too warm, refrigerate it for 15 or 20 minutes to firm it up a little.
- I find that sunflower seed butter has a milder, less noticeable flavor than tahini, but on the down side, it also has a tendency to turn baked goods green! It doesn't affect taste, just appearance, but that's something to keep in mind when deciding which one to use. The cookies pictured here are made with tahini. I didn't find the flavor to be too noticeable, but it does add a bit of nuttiness. That being said, taste the tahini before using to make sure you enjoy the flavor. Certain brands can be more bitter than others and that flavor will translate to the cookies.
- To make 2 flax eggs, whisk 2 tablespoons ground flax seed with 5 tablespoons water. Set aside for about 10 minutes to give the mixture time to gel.

Prep time: 10 minutes
Bake time: 10 minutes
Total time: 20 minutes
Yield: 12 cookies

- ¼ cup (50g) refined coconut oil, softened
- 3 tablespoons (48g) creamy peanut butter
- ½ cup (72g) coconut sugar
- 1 flax egg (see Tip) or 1 large egg, at room temperature
- 1 teaspoon pure vanilla extract
- 1¼ cups (124g) blanched almond flour
- ½ teaspoon sea salt
- ½ teaspoon baking soda
- ½ cup lightly crushed potato chips
- 2 ounces bittersweet chocolate, chopped, or chocolate chips (about ⅓ cup)
- ¼ cup lightly crushed pretzels
- ¼ cup roasted peanuts, roughly chopped
- Flaky sea salt, for sprinkling (optional)

Tip

To make a flax egg, whisk 1 tablespoon ground flax seed with 2½ tablespoons water. Set aside for about 10 minutes to give the mixture time to gel.

SWEET AND SALTY PEANUT BUTTER COOKIES

VEGAN • GLUTEN-FREE • DAIRY-FREE

You've got to trust me on this one. You may be side-eyeing me about putting potato chips and pretzels in your cookies, but if you're a fan of salty sweet things, you're going to *love* these. The chewy, decadent cookies are made with creamy peanut butter and have all sorts of delicious mix-ins: potato chips (I like using ones that have been fried in coconut oil), chocolate chunks, salted pretzels, and roasted peanuts. There is no shortage of crunchy, chewy textures. These are one of the few cookies that I'll say are best eaten cool instead of warm—when they're still warm, the potato chips and pretzels can be a little bit soft and chewy, but once the cookies are cooled, they go back to being crunchy.

PREHEAT the oven to 350°F; line a baking sheet with parchment paper.

IN a mixing bowl or bowl of a stand mixer fitted with the paddle attachment, mix the coconut oil, peanut butter, and coconut sugar until smooth. Add the egg and vanilla and mix until smooth.

ADD the almond flour, salt, and baking soda to the wet ingredients and stir until well incorporated. Fold in the potato chips, chopped chocolate, pretzels, and peanuts.

USE a large cookie scoop or spoon to form rounded cookies. Put them on the baking sheet and gently press to flatten slightly. Sprinkle with flaky sea salt, if desired. Bake for 10 to 12 minutes, until the cookies are golden brown around the edges.

LET the cookies cool on the baking sheet for 10 minutes before transferring to a wire rack to cool completely. I recommend waiting for these cookies to cool completely before eating for the best texture.

STORE in an airtight container at room temperature for up to 5 days.

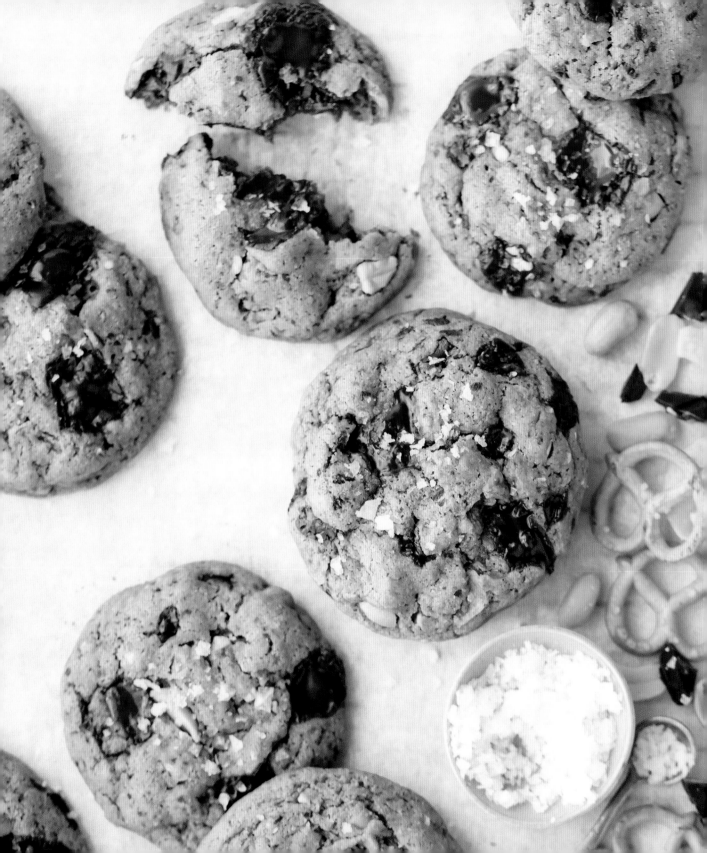

Prep time: 10 minutes

Chill time: 30 minutes

Bake time: 9 minutes

Total time: about 50 minutes

Yield: 12 cookies

FOR THE COOKIES

2 tablespoons refined coconut oil, slightly softened (see Tips)

2 tablespoons creamy almond butter

½ cup (72g) coconut sugar

1 flax egg (see Tips)

2 tablespoons organic molasses

½ teaspoon pure vanilla extract

½ teaspoon grated orange zest (optional)

1¼ cups (120g) blanched almond flour

1 teaspoon ground ginger

1 teaspoon ground cinnamon

¼ teaspoon ground nutmeg

½ teaspoon baking soda

¼ teaspoon kosher salt

FOR THE COATING

2 tablespoons coconut sugar

¼ teaspoon ground cinnamon

¼ teaspoon ground ginger

CHEWY GINGER COOKIES

PALEO • GRAIN-FREE • VEGAN • GLUTEN-FREE • DAIRY-FREE

These thin, crackled cookies quickly became a favorite as soon as I tasted them. The festive combination of molasses, orange zest, and warm spices makes one of the best holiday cookies I've tasted. The dough is rolled in a mixture of cinnamon, ginger, and coconut sugar, which creates a scrumptious crackly crust on each chewy cookie. Good luck having just one!

FOR THE COOKIES: In a large bowl, stir together the coconut oil, almond butter, and coconut sugar until fully combined, about 1 minute. Beat in the flax egg and then stir in the molasses, vanilla extract, and orange zest if using.

IN a separate bowl, whisk the almond flour with the ginger, cinnamon, nutmeg, baking soda, and salt. Add the dry ingredients to the molasses mixture and stir together until the dough is well mixed and comes together when pressed with your hands.

REFRIGERATE the dough for at least 30 minutes to make it easier to work with, or up to 48 hours.

WHEN you're ready to bake, preheat the oven to 350°F. Line a baking sheet with parchment paper.

FOR COATING THE COOKIES: Mix together the coconut sugar, cinnamon, and ginger in a small, shallow bowl.

USE a medium cookie scoop (mine holds about 1½ tablespoons of dough) or a spoon to make cookie dough balls. Roll each ball with your hands and then roll it in the coconut sugar mixture to coat. Put the cookies 2 inches apart on the baking sheet. Be sure to leave space between the cookies as they spread during baking.

BAKE for 9 to 11 minutes, until the cookies are light brown and a little darker around the edges. They may have cracks in them, which is to be expected. Let the cookies cool completely on the baking sheet before removing and serving. Store the cookies in an airtight container for up to 5 days.

Tips

- The coconut oil should be the consistency of softened butter. If it is supersoft or melted because the kitchen is too warm, refrigerate it for 15 to 30 minutes to firm it up slightly.
- To make a flax egg, mix 1 tablespoon ground flax seed with 2½ tablespoons water. Mix well and then set aside for 10 minutes to gel.

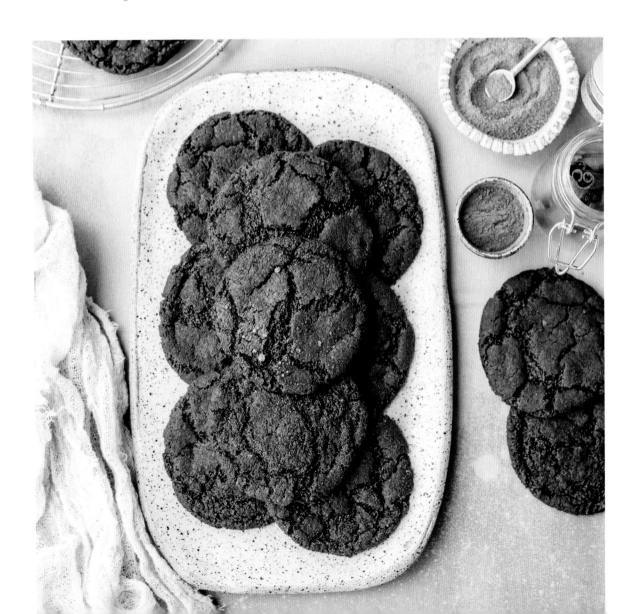

Prep time: 12 minutes

Bake time: 18 minutes

Total time: 30 minutes

Yield: 4 to 6 servings

⅓ cup (48g) coconut sugar

3 tablespoons coconut oil, softened (see Tips)

2 tablespoons smooth almond butter

1 flax egg (see Tips)

1 teaspoon pure vanilla extract

⅔ cup (64g) blanched almond flour

¼ cup (24g) cacao powder

¼ teaspoon baking soda

¼ teaspoon kosher salt

2 ounces bittersweet chocolate, chopped (about ⅓ cup)

Flaky sea salt (optional)

DOUBLE CHOCOLATE CHUNK SKILLET COOKIE

PALEO • GRAIN-FREE • VEGAN • GLUTEN-FREE • DAIRY-FREE

When you want a superrich, decadent, chocolate-loaded dessert, turn to this skillet cookie; you won't be disappointed. It's deeply chocolatey, with a chocolate dough loaded with chocolate chunks. Since it's baked in a small skillet, it's fun to serve to a small group of people. And it's definitely best when warm, though you can always warm it back up after it cools. I'd highly recommend using the flaky sea salt on top to help cut through the rich, deep chocolate flavor. For a peanut butter twist, use peanut butter instead of almond butter and swirl 2 tablespoons peanut butter into the cookie dough before baking. A scoop of ice cream and a drizzle of Hot Fudge Sauce (page 279) make this even better!

PREHEAT the oven to 350°F. Lightly grease a 6½-inch cast-iron skillet or two or three 3-inch ramekins with coconut oil.

IN a mixing bowl, whisk the coconut sugar with the coconut oil and almond butter until combined, about 1 minute. Add the flax egg and vanilla extract and mix until smooth.

ADD the almond flour, cacao powder, baking soda, and salt to the wet ingredients and mix until smooth. Fold in the chopped chocolate.

PRESS the dough into the prepared skillet and sprinkle with flaky sea salt, if desired.

BAKE for 16 to 18 minutes, staying closer to 16 minutes for a gooier cookie or closer to 18 for a firmer cookie. Let the cookie cool for 5 minutes in the skillet set on a wire rack and then serve from the skillet, warm or cooled.

REMOVE any leftover skillet cookie from the pan and refrigerate, well wrapped in plastic wrap, for up to 5 days.

Tips

- The coconut oil should be the texture of soft butter. If it liquefies because the kitchen is too warm, refrigerate for 15 or 20 minutes.
- To make a flax egg, mix 1 tablespoon ground flax seed with 2½ tablespoons water. Stir well and then let the mixture sit for about 10 minutes to gel.
- If you want to prepare this in advance and bake it later, wrap the skillet, filled with the dough, with plastic wrap and refrigerate for up to 24 hours.

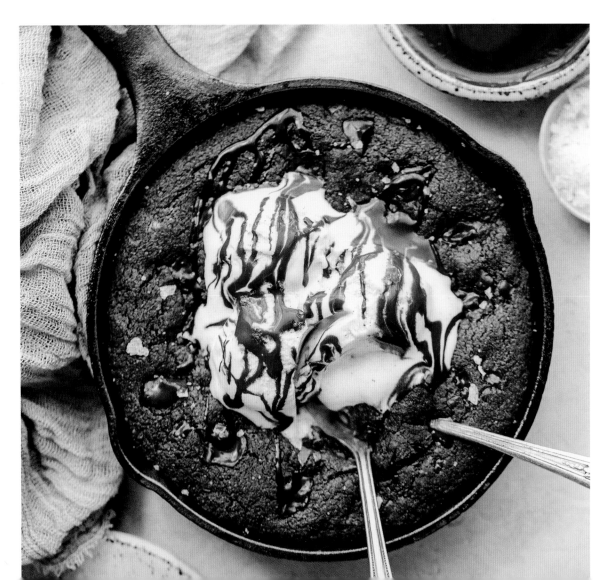

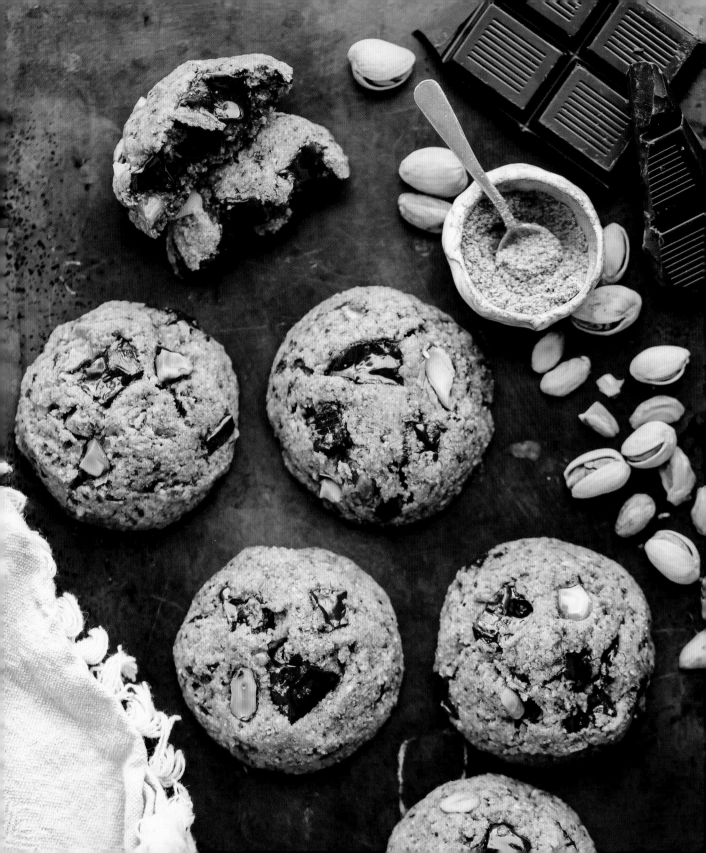

DARK CHOCOLATE, PISTACHIO, AND CARDAMOM COOKIES

PALEO • GRAIN-FREE • VEGAN • GLUTEN-FREE • DAIRY-FREE

I can't get over these cookies! They're so soft and flavorful, and unique enough to have you inquisitively taking your second, then third bite, letting the flavors dance on your tongue. The first time I tested them I couldn't stop breaking off pieces, until three cookies were gone when they hadn't been out of the oven for more than an hour. Oops. The crunch of the pistachio pairs beautifully with the fragrant citrusy notes of the cardamom, while the chocolate adds a sumptuous richness. Because these are vegan and made with a flax egg, they stay incredibly soft and thick. Dip in a cup of almond milk, pistachio milk, or a warm cup of tea and prepare to be transported into cookie heaven!

Prep time: 10 minutes
Chill time: 1 hour
Bake time: 10 minutes
Total time: 1 hour 20 minutes
Yield: 13 to 15 cookies

⅔ cup (96g) coconut sugar

½ cup (100g) refined coconut oil, slightly softened (see Tips)

1 flax egg (see Tips)

1 teaspoon pure vanilla extract

2¼ cups (216g) blanched almond flour

1 teaspoon ground cardamom

½ teaspoon baking soda

½ teaspoon kosher salt

4 ounces bittersweet chocolate, chopped (about ⅔ cup), plus extra for decoration, if desired

¼ cup shelled pistachios, chopped, plus extra for decoration, if desired

IN the bowl of a stand mixer fitted with the paddle attachment or in a mixing bowl, beat the coconut sugar and coconut oil on medium speed until fluffy. Add the flax egg and vanilla and mix until nicely blended. If you prefer, you can stir the ingredients in a mixing bowl with a sturdy spoon.

ADD the almond flour, cardamom, baking soda, and salt to the wet ingredients and, with the mixer on medium-low, mix until well incorporated, or mix the ingredients in by hand. Fold in the chopped chocolate and pistachios.

COVER the bowl with plastic wrap and refrigerate for at least 1 hour, or up to 24 hours. This chilling time lets the flavors meld and the cardamom flavor permeate the dough.

PREHEAT the oven to 350°F. Line a baking sheet with parchment paper.

USE a medium cookie scoop that holds about 1½ ounces of dough to form cookies. You can also use a spoon to form rounded mounds of dough. Put them about 2 inches apart on the prepared baking sheet. If desired, press more chocolate chunks, pistachios, or both

CONTINUES

169

onto the top of the cookies (I do this to make them look pretty!). Bake for 10 to 12 minutes, until the cookies are just beginning to turn golden brown around the edges.

LET the cookies cool for 10 minutes on the baking sheet and then move them to a wire rack to cool completely. Store the cookies in an airtight container on the counter for 3 days, or in the refrigerator for up to 1 week.

Tips

- The coconut oil should be the consistency of softened butter. If it is supersoft or melted because the kitchen is too warm, refrigerate it for 15 to 30 minutes to firm it up slightly.
- To make a flax egg, whisk 1 tablespoon ground flax seed with 2½ tablespoons water. Set aside for about 10 minutes to give the mixture time to gel.

ICED OATMEAL COOKIES

VEGAN • GLUTEN-FREE • DAIRY-FREE

These oatmeal cookies remind me of afternoons after school, tearing open a package of iced oatmeal cookies that were crisp and buttery with a touch of sweet icing. With a little more chew and a lot less preservatives, these will bring back memories of stacking cookies and enjoying them after a quick dunk in milk. My version is chewier and so buttery, thanks to the coconut oil and cashew butter, and the simple icing drizzle makes them irresistible. Store in the fridge for the best chewy cookie texture and snappy icing!

FOR THE COOKIES: In a large bowl, mix together the coconut oil and coconut sugar until fully combined and resembles wet sand. Stir in the cashew butter and vanilla extract, followed by the egg. Keep mixing until the dough is blended.

IN another bowl, whisk together the oats, almond flour, baking powder, baking soda, and salt. Add to the wet ingredients and stir until fully mixed.

COVER the cookie dough with plastic wrap and refrigerate for at least 2 hours, or up to 3 days.

WHEN you're ready to bake, preheat the oven to 350°F. Line 2 baking sheets with parchment paper.

USE a small cookie scoop or spoon to scoop out dough balls and arrange them about 2 inches apart on the baking sheets. With the palm of your hand, press gently on the cookie balls so that they are about 1½ inches in diameter.

ONE baking sheet at a time, bake the cookies in the center of the oven for about 12 minutes, or until just pale gold. Let the cookies cool completely on the baking sheets before transferring them to wire racks set on parchment paper.

FOR THE GLAZE: Whisk together the coconut butter and maple syrup. The mixture may seize up, but the milk will thin it back out. Whisk in the warmed milk, a tablespoon at a time, until the glaze

Prep time: 15 minutes
Chill time: 2 hours 30 minutes
Bake time: 24 minutes
Total time: about 3¼ hours
Yield: about 17 cookies

FOR THE COOKIES
⅓ cup (67g) refined coconut oil, slightly softened (see Tips)

⅔ cup (96g) coconut sugar

¼ cup (64g) cashew butter

1 teaspoon pure vanilla extract

1 flax egg (see Tips) or 1 large egg, at room temperature

¾ cup (72g) gluten-free rolled oats

1 cup plus 2 tablespoons (108g) blanched almond flour

½ teaspoon baking powder

½ teaspoon baking soda

½ teaspoon kosher salt

FOR THE GLAZE
¼ cup coconut butter, melted

1 tablespoon pure maple syrup

Up to 4 tablespoons dairy-free milk, such as unsweetened almond milk, warmed in the microwave

CONTINUES

is smooth and thin enough to drizzle. (It takes me about 3 tablespoons, but could be a little bit more or less for you.)

USE a spoon to drizzle the glaze over the cookies, letting excess glaze drip onto the parchment paper. Transfer to the refrigerator for at least 30 minutes to let the glaze set.

Tips

- The coconut oil should be the consistency of softened butter. If it is supersoft or melted because the kitchen is too warm, refrigerate it for 15 to 30 minutes to firm it up.
- To make a flax egg, mix 1 tablespoon ground flax seed with 2½ tablespoons water. Stir well and then let the mixture sit for about 10 minutes to gel.

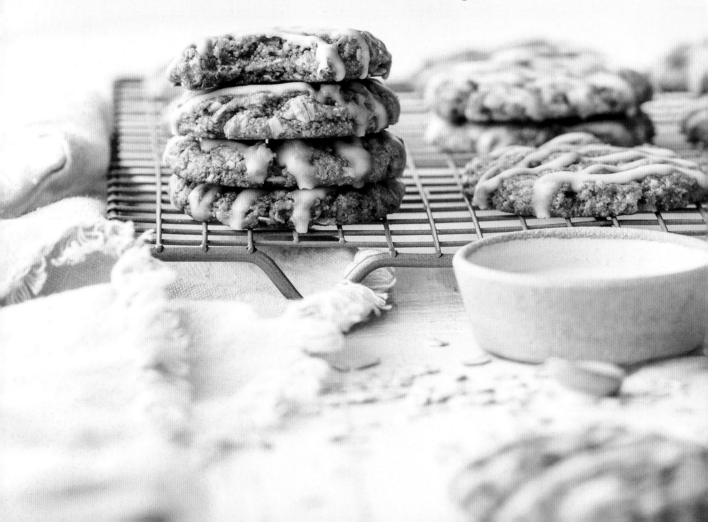

HOMEMADE GRAHAM CRACKERS

PALEO • GRAIN-FREE • VEGAN • GLUTEN-FREE • DAIRY-FREE

As I was testing recipes for this book, I was taking treats with me whenever I went to meet up with friends to get feedback on my creations. One day I went to lunch with my friend Jill and among the treats were some Paleo Vanilla-Bean Marshmallows (page 245) and a Homemade Chocolate Bar (page 231). Soon after lunch she sent me a video message formally requesting that the book also include homemade graham crackers so completely homemade Paleo s'mores could be had. So here we have them: graham crackers, just like you remember, crunchy and barely sweetened, with a hint of cinnamon. Perfect for s'mores.

IN a mixing bowl, whisk the almond flour with the coconut flour, tapioca flour, coconut sugar, baking powder, cinnamon, and salt to get out all of the clumps and incorporate fully.

IN a separate microwave-safe bowl, combine the maple syrup, coconut oil, and milk. Microwave for 30 seconds and then stir until the coconut oil is fully melted. Repeat the process if necessary.

ADD the liquid ingredients to the dry ingredients and stir until all the dry ingredients are moistened and the dough comes together when gently pressed. It may seem like there's not enough moisture, but keep mixing and it will all come together.

PUT the dough on a sheet of parchment paper or a silicone baking mat. Press it into a rectangle and top with another sheet of parchment. With the dough between the sheets of parchment, roll it into a rectangle measuring approximately 10 × 12½ inches and about ⅛ inch thick. If the crackers are too thick, they won't be crunchy enough. If necessary, trim the edges and fill in any gaps around the sides and then reroll to smooth out the dough. One of the perks of gluten-free baking is that the dough won't toughen from rerolling!

Prep time: 45 minutes
Chill time: 1 hour
Bake time: 10 minutes
Total time: about 2 hours
Yield: 20 crackers

1½ cups (144g) blanched almond flour

2 tablespoons coconut flour

2 tablespoons tapioca flour

2 tablespoons coconut sugar

1 teaspoon baking powder

1 teaspoon ground cinnamon

¼ teaspoon kosher salt

2 tablespoons pure maple syrup

2 tablespoons refined coconut oil, softened

1 tablespoon dairy-free milk, such as unsweetened almond or coconut milk

Tip

Leftovers? Pulse crackers in a food processor to make graham cracker crumbs and use for pie crusts and parfaits, or sprinkle on top of other desserts as a garnish.

CONTINUES

USING a ruler and sharp knife or pizza cutter, cut the dough into 2½-inch squares, for a total of 20 squares. Lay the squares slightly separated from each other on a parchment-lined baking sheet.

WITHOUT cutting through the dough squares, run a knife or pizza cutter lightly down the center of each square to resemble how the halves of a graham cracker look. Poke the dough with a fork, again making sure not to press all the way through.

TRANSFER to the refrigerator and let chill for 1 hour. After an hour, preheat the oven to 350°F.

BAKE the crackers for 10 to 12 minutes, until light golden brown. They'll feel a little soft when they first come out of the oven, but they'll firm up as they cool on the baking sheet. Lift the cooled crackers off the baking sheet.

STORE the graham crackers in an airtight bag or container. For the crispiest graham crackers, enjoy in the first 3 days after baking.

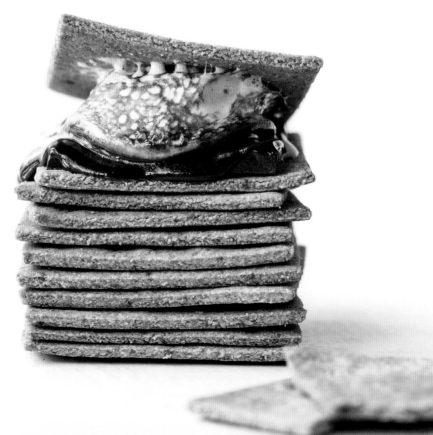

CRANBERRY-ORANGE PISTACHIO COOKIES

PALEO • GRAIN-FREE • VEGAN • GLUTEN-FREE • DAIRY-FREE

These bright, tender cookies are the perfect holiday cookie when you need a little break from the chocolate and caramel decadence of the holidays, but still want something that's festive and mouthwateringly delicious. A bit of honey adds a floral sweetness that plays well with freshly grated orange zest and cinnamon, while the chewy cranberries and crunchy, buttery pistachios add scrumptious texture. The sprinkling of raw turbinado sugar on top makes them sparkle—perfect for any holiday cookie platter (or any other day of the year)!

PREHEAT the oven to 350°F. Line one large or two smaller baking sheets with parchment paper.

IN a mixing bowl or a stand mixer fitted with the paddle attachment, beat the coconut oil and coconut sugar until fully combined and a little fluffy. Add the honey, egg, orange zest, and vanilla and mix well.

IN a separate bowl, whisk the almond flour with the baking soda, cinnamon, and salt. Add the dry ingredients to the wet ingredients and mix until fully incorporated with no dry streaks left. Fold in the pistachios and dried cranberries. (If you want to bake the cookies later, cover the bowl with plastic wrap and refrigerate for up to 24 hours.)

USE a medium cookie scoop (mine holds about 1½ tablespoons) or spoon to scoop rounded cookies and put them on the baking sheet(s). Leave about 2 inches between each cookie as they spread during baking. Top the cookies with extra pistachios and raw turbinado sugar, if desired.

CONTINUES

Prep time: 15 minutes
Bake time: 10 or 20 minutes
Total time: 25 or 35 minutes
Yield: 18 cookies

- ½ cup (100g) refined coconut oil, softened (see Tips)
- ¼ cup (36g) coconut sugar
- 3 tablespoons honey or pure maple syrup (maple syrup keeps them vegan)
- 1 flax egg (see Tips) or 1 large egg, at room temperature
- Grated zest of 1 orange
- ½ teaspoon pure vanilla extract
- 2½ cups (240g) blanched almond flour
- 1¼ teaspoons baking soda
- 1 teaspoon ground cinnamon
- ¼ teaspoon sea salt
- ½ cup chopped shelled pistachios, plus extra for garnish
- ¼ cup roughly chopped dried cranberries (see Tips)
- 1 to 2 tablespoons raw turbinado sugar, for garnish (optional)

BAKE one sheet of cookies for about 10 minutes, until the cookies' edges are set and golden brown. Let the cookies cool on the baking sheet for about 10 minutes and then transfer to a wire rack to cool completely. Repeat with the second baking sheet if you used two sheets.

STORE the cookies in an airtight container at room temperature for up to 3 days, or in the refrigerator for up to a week. I prefer these refrigerated!

Tips

- The coconut oil should be the consistency of softened butter. If it is supersoft or melted because the kitchen is too warm, refrigerate it for 15 to 30 minutes to firm it up slightly.
- To make a flax egg, mix 1 tablespoon ground flax seed with 2½ tablespoons water. Stir well and then let the mixture sit for about 10 minutes to gel.
- I always seek out dried cranberries that are sweetened with apple juice instead of cane sugar. My favorite brand is Made in Nature.

COCONUT-DATE MACAROONS

PALEO • GRAIN-FREE • VEGAN • NO-BAKE • GLUTEN-FREE • DAIRY-FREE

Dates are magical little fruits. They may be brown and shriveled in appearance, but they are full of caramel-y sweetness and are delightfully chewy and sticky when you bite into one. In this recipe, they provide all the sweetening and all the sticking power needed to make coconut macaroons and add their own sumptuous flavor to the mix. The macaroons are dipped and drizzled in chocolate and sprinkled with an extra bit of flaky salt to help cut through the sweetness of the date caramel. If you're a fan of dates and macaroons, these just might be your dream come true! Something to keep in mind as not all dates are created equal: Make sure you get your hands on fresh, plump dates. If they're dried out, they won't blend into the luscious caramel-like paste we're after. If your dates feel a little bit dry, soak them in hot water for 10 to 15 minutes before using to plump them back up.

Prep time: 15 minutes
Chill time: 30 minutes
Total time: 45 minutes
Yield: 14 to 16 macaroons

1 cup (about 8 large) roughly chopped pitted Medjool dates

½ cup hot tap water

3 tablespoons refined coconut oil, softened

½ teaspoon kosher salt

2½ cups unsweetened flaked coconut

4 ounces bittersweet chocolate, finely chopped (about ⅔ cup)

1 teaspoon flaky sea salt, or more if necessary

LINE a baking sheet with parchment paper.

IN a high-powered blender (I use a Vitamix) or bowl of a food processor fitted with the metal blade, combine the pitted dates, hot water, coconut oil, and kosher salt. Blend until a thick, caramel-y paste forms, scraping down the sides of the blender or bowl of the food processor to ensure that the dates blend completely. If you don't have a blender, stir the ingredients with a sturdy spoon until paste-like.

IF the coconut flakes are on the large size, chop them until small. Put the coconut in a mixing bowl. Scrape the date mixture over the coconut and stir to combine until the coconut is completely mixed in.

USE a small cookie scoop or spoon to form about 15 cookies. Put them on the prepared baking sheet and transfer to the refrigerator for about 30 minutes to firm up.

IN a small microwave-safe bowl, microwave the chocolate for 1 minute. Stir, and then continue to melt in 15-second intervals,

CONTINUES

stirring between each, until the chocolate is fully melted. (You might need to do this five or six times; the chocolate won't melt completely but will liquefy when stirred.)

ONCE the macaroons are firm, dip the bottom of each in the melted chocolate, gently scraping any excess chocolate off the bottom, and return each macaroon to the parchment-lined baking sheet. Drizzle with the remaining chocolate using a small whisk, fork, or piping bag.

SPRINKLE the flaky sea salt on top of the cookies and return to the refrigerator to firm up the chocolate.

STORE the macaroons in an airtight container in the refrigerator for up to 1 week, or in the freezer for up to 1 month.

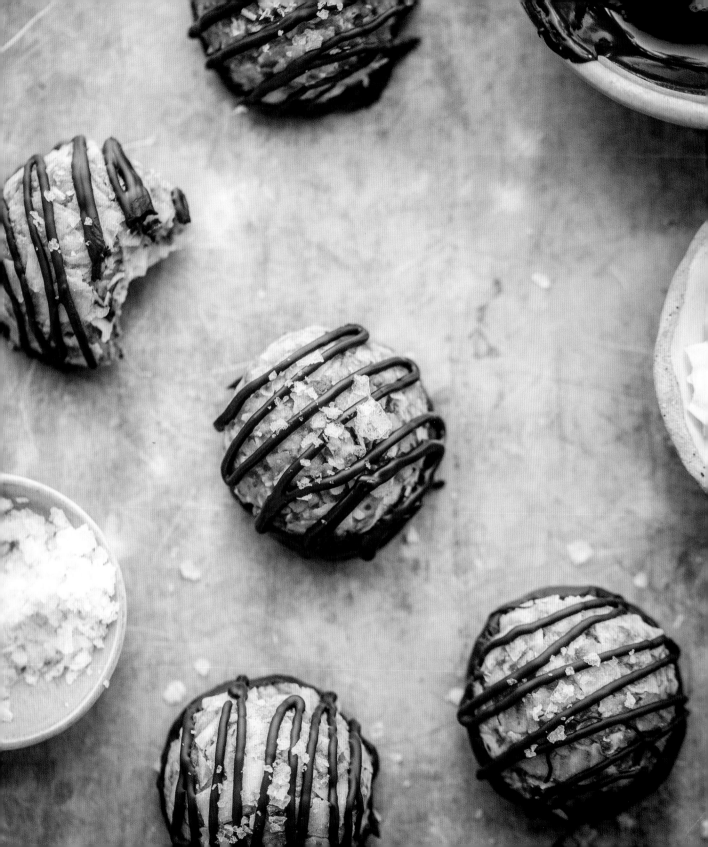

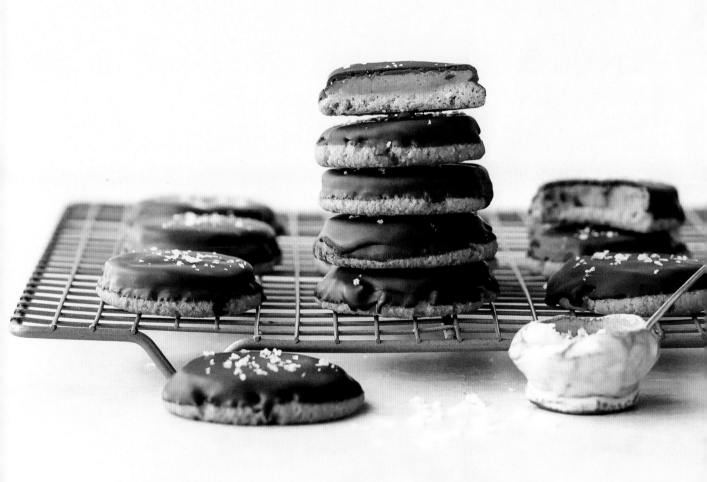

CHOCOLATE-DIPPED PEANUT BUTTER SHORTBREAD COOKIES

GRAIN-FREE • VEGAN • GLUTEN-FREE • DAIRY-FREE

When I was a first grader, my friends and I joined the Girl Scout troop at my school. Being a sweet-toothed kid, I couldn't wait to get my hands on those cookies. As many as I sold to others, I asked my parents to match and buy us a bunch of my favorites to store in the freezer to have all year round. Being the chocolate–peanut butter addict that I was (and still am), I always wanted the chocolate-covered peanut butter shortbread cookies. Luckily, I am able to re-create my favorite cookie, keeping it gluten-free, grain-free, and vegan. It satisfies those crunchy, peanut butter-y cravings I have. If you want, you can scrape the peanut butter off the top of the cookie with your teeth, the way I always did as a kid.

LINE a baking sheet with parchment paper.

FOR THE COOKIES: In a mixing bowl or bowl of a stand mixer fitted with the paddle attachment, whisk together the almond flour, arrowroot starch, and salt. Add the maple syrup, coconut oil, and vanilla and mix until combined.

SHAPE about 2 teaspoons of the dough into a flattened round, about 2 inches across and ¼ inch thick, and set on the baking sheet. Repeat with the remaining dough to make about 15 cookies. Refrigerate for at least 30 minutes, or up to 24 hours.

WHEN you're ready to bake, preheat the oven to 325°F.

BAKE the cookies for 20 to 22 minutes, until golden brown around the edges. The longer you bake them, the crispier they'll be, so watch them carefully. If you like crispy cookies, make sure they don't overbake. Remove the cookies from the oven and let them cool completely on the baking sheet.

FOR THE PEANUT BUTTER FILLING: In a mixing bowl, stir together the peanut butter, maple syrup, coconut flour, and salt, if

Prep time: 20 minutes
Chill time: 40 minutes
Bake time: 20 minutes
Total time: 1 hour 20 minutes
Yield: 15 cookies

FOR THE COOKIES

1 cup (96g) blanched almond flour

¼ cup (32g) arrowroot starch

⅛ teaspoon kosher salt

3 tablespoons (63g) pure maple syrup

2 tablespoons refined coconut oil, melted

½ teaspoon pure vanilla extract

FOR THE PEANUT BUTTER FILLING

⅔ cup creamy peanut butter

2 tablespoons pure maple syrup

1 tablespoon coconut flour

½ teaspoon kosher salt (skip if the peanut butter is salted, or add to taste)

FOR THE CHOCOLATE DIP

3 ounces bittersweet chocolate, chopped or in chips (about ½ cup)

2 teaspoons softened coconut oil or cacao butter

Flaky sea salt, for garnish (optional)

CONTINUES

using. Scoop out a 2-teaspoon-sized ball of this mixture and press it gently into the center of a cooled cookie. Leave a narrow rim around the cookie's edges. Flatten the filling on top of the cookie using your fingertips. Repeat with the remaining cookies and filling.

FOR THE CHOCOLATE COATING: Once the cookies are fully cooled and have the peanut butter on top, combine the chocolate and coconut oil in a small microwave-safe bowl. Microwave for 1 minute and then stir the mixture. The chocolate will be soft but not fluid. It should become smooth as you stir it—but if not, microwave for another 30 seconds and stir again until smooth, fluid, and satiny.

DIP the top of a cookie into the chocolate, covering the peanut butter. Let the excess chocolate drip off and then return the cookie to the parchment-lined baking sheet, chocolate side up. Repeat until all the cookies are coated. Sprinkle with flaky sea salt, if desired.

REFRIGERATE the cookies for at least 10 minutes to firm up the chocolate and then serve.

STORE in an airtight container in the refrigerator for up to 1 week, or in the freezer for up to 3 months.

SNICKERDOODLES

PALEO • GRAIN-FREE • VEGAN • GLUTEN-FREE • DAIRY-FREE

I'm going to make a confession: Snickerdoodles were never my favorite cookie. I've always preferred something with chocolate and/or peanut butter in it, but that does not mean that I can't appreciate a great snickerdoodle. What makes a snickerdoodle great? It must be soft—crunchy snickerdoodles just don't do the trick; we need soft, chewy, tender cookies. They also have to have cinnamon flavor laced all the way through, including as part of the sugary coating. Cream of tartar is another must: It helps to create that classic snickerdoodle flavor, the signature snickerdoodle tang, while also contributing to the chewy texture. These snickerdoodles check all the boxes and are beloved by many snickerdoodle fans who adore their soft texture and spiced and sugared coating! They're also ready in a snap—no refrigerating the dough needed!

FOR THE COOKIES: Preheat the oven to 350°F. Line a baking sheet with a silicone mat or parchment paper.

IN a mixing bowl, stir together the almond flour, coconut flour, baking soda, cream of tartar, salt, and cinnamon. Add the coconut oil, maple syrup, and vanilla and stir until thoroughly combined.

FOR THE CINNAMON SUGAR: In a separate small bowl, stir together the coconut sugar and cinnamon.

USING a cookie scoop or spoon, measure about 1 heaping tablespoon dough and roll it into a ball. Roll the ball in the cinnamon sugar mixture. Repeat with the rest of the dough and cinnamon sugar.

PUT the coated dough balls on the prepared baking sheet about 2 inches apart. Flatten the dough slightly with your palm or the flat bottom of a glass; they won't spread much during baking but should not touch. Bake for about 10 minutes, until light golden brown. Make sure not to overbake to keep the cookies soft and chewy.

Prep time: 10 minutes
Bake time: 10 minutes
Total time: 20 minutes
Yield: 24 cookies

FOR THE COOKIES
1¾ cups (168g) blanched almond flour
¼ cup (32g) coconut flour
½ teaspoon baking soda
½ teaspoon cream of tartar
½ teaspoon kosher salt
½ teaspoon ground cinnamon
⅓ cup (67g) refined coconut oil, melted
⅓ cup (113g) pure maple syrup
1 tablespoon pure vanilla extract

FOR THE CINNAMON SUGAR
¼ cup coconut sugar
1 tablespoon ground cinnamon

CONTINUES

LET the snickerdoodles cool for about 10 minutes on the baking sheet and then transfer to a wire rack to cool completely.

STORE in an airtight container at room temperature for up to 5 days. For a chewier texture, store in the refrigerator.

Tip

To add some variety to these cookies, vary the spices that the cookies are rolled in. One of my favorite options is a chai snickerdoodle. Use a combination of 1 teaspoon cinnamon, ½ teaspoon nutmeg, ½ teaspoon ground ginger, ⅛ teaspoon ground cardamom, and a pinch of black pepper in place of the cinnamon in the cinnamon sugar mixture.

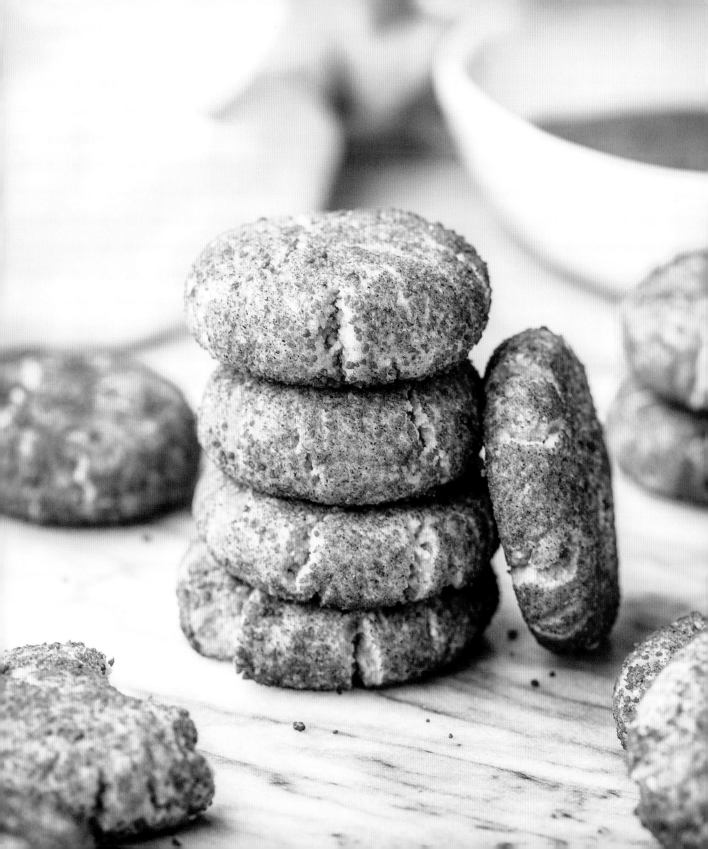

Prep time: 10 minutes
Chill time: 1 hour
Bake time: 11 minutes
Total time: 1 hour 20 minutes
Yield: 18 cookies

½ cup (100g) refined coconut oil, melted

¾ cup (183g) canned pure pumpkin puree (see Tips)

¾ cup (108g) coconut sugar

1 flax egg (see Tips)

2 teaspoons pure vanilla extract

1 teaspoon baking powder

1 teaspoon baking soda

2 teaspoons ground cinnamon

½ teaspoon nutmeg

¼ teaspoon ground cloves

½ teaspoon kosher salt

1 cup (96g) blanched almond flour

⅓ cup plus 1 tablespoon (50g) coconut flour

6 ounces bittersweet chocolate chunks

SOFT PUMPKIN-CHOCOLATE CHIP COOKIES

PALEO • GRAIN-FREE • VEGAN • GLUTEN-FREE • DAIRY-FREE

If you've ever dreamt of a treat that's half chocolate chip cookie and half warmly spiced pumpkin bread, then you've found the right recipe. These soft chocolate chip cookies are a pumpkin lover's dream. They're soft and cakey, thanks to the pumpkin puree, and warmly spiced from the cinnamon, nutmeg, and cloves that are laced throughout the dough. The scent of the cookies baking will make your mouth water, so don't resist trying one warm—the melty chocolate and fragrant spices are perfect with a coffee, chai latte, or cup of tea.

IN a large mixing bowl, combine the melted coconut oil, pumpkin puree, coconut sugar, flax egg, and vanilla. Whisk until well mixed and completely smooth. Add the baking powder, baking soda, cinnamon, nutmeg, cloves, and salt. Stir well and then add the almond flour and coconut flour. Stir until a smooth dough forms and the dry ingredients are completely incorporated. Fold in the chocolate chunks.

CHILL the dough, covered in plastic wrap, for at least 1 hour, or up to 24 hours. Don't skip this step. The dough needs to chill so that the coconut oil can firm up and prevent the cookies from spreading too much.

WHEN you're ready to bake, preheat the oven to 350°F. Line two baking sheets with parchment paper.

USING a large cookie scoop or spoon, scoop about 18 mounds of dough onto the baking sheets, leaving 2 inches between the cookies. Press down slightly. Bake for 11 to 14 minutes, until crispy around the edges. Let the cookies cool on the baking sheets for about 10 minutes before transferring to a wire rack to cool completely.

STORE in an airtight container at room temperature for up to 5 days.

Tips

- Use a thick, unseasoned pumpkin puree here, not one that is watery or liquidy. If it is, you may want to cook it down in a saucepan over medium-low heat for 5 to 10 minutes, stirring frequently, to help some of the water evaporate. Cool before using.
- To make the flax egg, whisk 2 tablespoons ground flax seed with 2½ tablespoons water. Let stand for 10 minutes to gel.

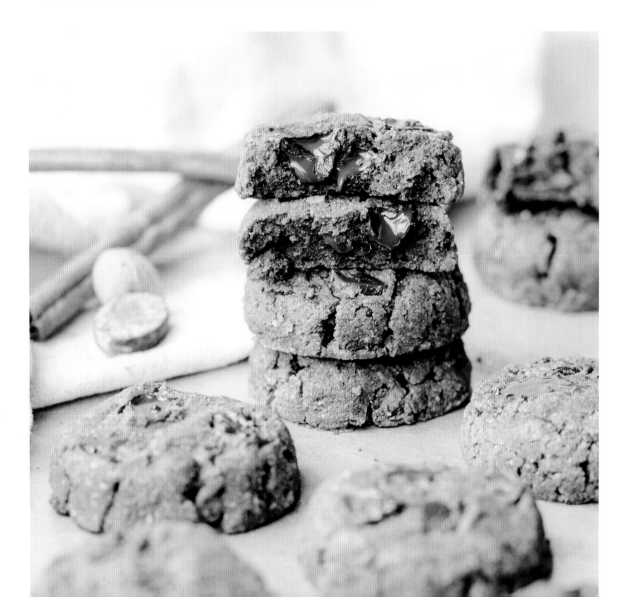

CHAPTER FIVE

Brownies and Bars

A FEW TIPS AND TRICKS FOR SUCCESS:

Bars are one of the best types of desserts to make ahead and store in the freezer so they're ready in a flash when you need them. All of the recipes in this chapter freeze well when they're wrapped well in plastic or beeswax wrap and kept in an airtight container.

To easily remove bars and brownies from their pans, line the pans with parchment paper! I do this by cutting the parchment paper sheet to the shape of the pan (usually a square) and then cutting a slit (about 4 inches) in from each corner toward the center. Then I place the parchment in the pan and press down so it nestles into it. This makes it super easy to take the bars out of the pan when they're ready to be cut!

For the easiest slicing, I recommend letting the bars chill in the refrigerator for at least an hour before removing them from the pan to cut, and using a sharp knife. This will give you the most even squares.

For the chewiest brownies and blondies, underbake them slightly. Overbaking will result in a dry bar. I make all my bars in an 8 × 8-inch pan. If you want more servings, double the recipe and bake in a 13 × 9-inch pan.

Prep time: 15 minutes
Bake time: 16 minutes
Total time: about 30 minutes
Yield: 16 brownies

FOR THE BROWNIES

1 teaspoon instant espresso powder

2 tablespoons boiling water

2 ounces (57g) unsweetened chocolate, chopped (about ⅓ cup)

2 tablespoons refined coconut oil, melted

½ cup (128g) creamy natural almond butter

⅓ cup (48g) coconut sugar

3 tablespoons (63g) pure maple syrup

1 flax egg (see Tip) or 1 large egg, at room temperature

1 teaspoon pure vanilla extract

⅓ cup (32g) blanched almond flour

½ cup (48g) cacao powder

2 teaspoons ground cinnamon

¾ teaspoon baking soda

½ teaspoon fine sea salt

¼ teaspoon cayenne pepper powder

3 ounces bittersweet chocolate, chopped or as chips (about 6 tablespoons)

FOR THE GANACHE

4 ounces bittersweet chocolate, chopped or as chips (about ⅔ cup)

¼ cup canned full-fat coconut milk

MEXICAN CHOCOLATE BROWNIES

PALEO • GRAIN-FREE • VEGAN • GLUTEN-FREE • DAIRY-FREE

When I was in the middle of recipe testing for this book, I took a road trip to Santa Fe, New Mexico. I was sitting in a small chocolate shop, sipping on a mug of the most delectable, lightly spiced hot chocolate—it had the warmth of cinnamon mixed with a little tingle of cayenne that lingered on my tongue after the chocolate had melted down my throat. I knew I had to re-create those flavors, and when I got home from that trip Mexican chocolate brownies were born. The rich and fudgy brownies start with deep chocolate flavor and finish with a linger of cayenne on the back of your tongue.

PREHEAT the oven to 350°F. Line an 8 × 8-inch baking pan with parchment paper and grease lightly with coconut oil.

FOR THE BROWNIES: In a small bowl, whisk the espresso powder with the boiling water.

PUT the unsweetened chocolate and coconut oil in a microwave-safe container and microwave for 30 seconds. Stir and repeat until the chocolate and coconut oil are completely melted and smooth. Add the diluted espresso, almond butter, coconut sugar, and maple syrup and whisk until completely combined. Whisk in the egg and vanilla.

IN a separate bowl, whisk the almond flour with the cacao powder, cinnamon, baking soda, sea salt, and cayenne pepper. Add the dry ingredients to the chocolate mixture and fold until completely combined. Stir in the chopped chocolate or chips. Spread the batter in the prepared pan, making it as even as you can.

BAKE for 16 to 18 minutes, until only a few crumbs are attached when a toothpick is inserted into the center but it's not too wet. Remove the brownies from the oven and let cool in the pan set on a wire rack.

FOR THE GANACHE: Put the chocolate in a small, heat-proof bowl. In another bowl, heat the coconut milk in the microwave for 45 seconds, or until hot and steaming. Pour the hot milk over the chocolate and let the ganache stand for about 2 minutes. Whisk until smooth and the chocolate melts. Spread the ganache over the cooled brownies.

LET the ganache cool completely before cutting and serving the brownies. I like to refrigerate them overnight before cutting for cleaner cuts.

STORE in an airtight container at room temperature for 2 to 3 days, or in the refrigerator for up to 1 week.

Tip

To make a flax egg, mix 1 tablespoon ground flax seed with 2½ tablespoons water. Whisk well and then set aside at room temperature for about 10 minutes to gel.

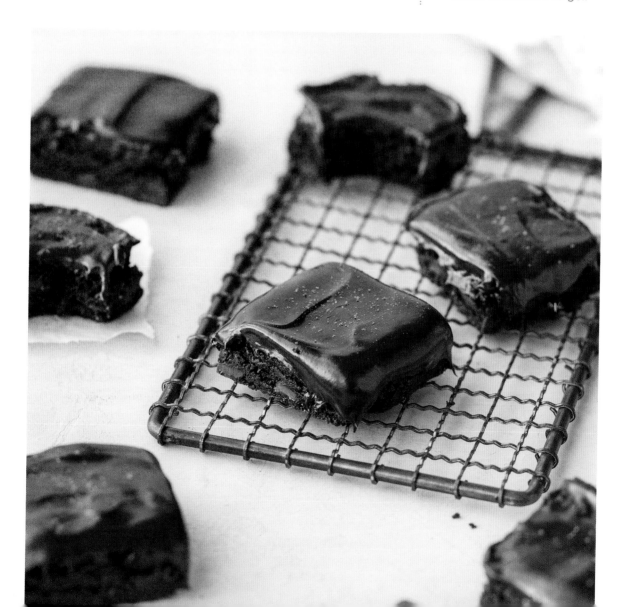

Prep time: 20 minutes
Bake time: 50 minutes
Total time: 1 hour and 10 minutes
Yield: 16 bars

FOR THE CRUST AND CRUMBLE

1¾ cups (168g) blanched almond flour

1 cup (96g) gluten-free rolled oats

¼ cup (32g) coconut flour

½ teaspoon ground cinnamon

¼ teaspoon kosher salt

⅓ cup (113g) pure maple syrup

⅓ cup (67g) refined coconut oil, softened (see Tip)

¼ cup (64g) cashew butter or almond butter

FOR THE SPICED STONE-FRUIT FILLING

1 pound mixed stone fruits, such as plums, peaches, and nectarines, pitted and chopped into 1-inch cubes (no need to peel, unless that's what you prefer)

3 tablespoons coconut sugar

2 tablespoons tapioca flour

1 teaspoon pure vanilla extract

1½ teaspoons ground cinnamon

1 teaspoon ground ginger

1 teaspoon ground cardamom

¼ teaspoon allspice

SPICED STONE-FRUIT CRUMBLE BARS

VEGAN • GLUTEN-FREE • DAIRY-FREE

One of my favorite times of the year is late summer, when a stroll through the farmers' market on a warm day smells like fresh strawberries and ripe peaches. I'm always drawn toward the rainbow-colored tables covered in piles of plums, pluots, nectarines, peaches, and apricots. There's nothing better than sinking your teeth into a ripe nectarine and letting the juice drip down your chin . . . but these stone fruit bars come a close second. When you've had your fill of fresh stone fruit (or just want to switch it up), cut some of them up, toss with a little sweetener and some warm spices, and bake until golden and bubbly between an oat-based crust that doubles as a crumble topping. The cinnamon, ginger, cardamom, and allspice add an extra layer of delectableness that will make your mouth water!

PREHEAT the oven to 350°F. Line an 8 × 8-inch metal baking pan with parchment paper and grease lightly with coconut oil.

FOR THE CRUST AND CRUMBLE: In a mixing bowl, combine the almond flour, rolled oats, coconut flour, cinnamon, and salt. Whisk to combine. Add the maple syrup, coconut oil, and cashew butter. Stir until the dry ingredients are completely moistened, sticky, and still a little crumbly. Measure out 1 cup and refrigerate to use later as the crumble topping.

PRESS the rest of the dough evenly into the bottom of the pan, using your hands, a spatula, or the back of a spoon to make an even layer.

BAKE the crust for about 10 minutes, until set and lightly browned. Set aside to cool in the pan set on a wire rack.

FOR THE FILLING: In a medium saucepan, mix together the cubed stone fruit, coconut sugar, tapioca flour, vanilla, cinnamon, ginger, cardamom, and allspice. Simmer gently over low heat for about 10 minutes, stirring occasionally and scraping up the bottom to make sure nothing burns. Remove the saucepan from the heat.

SPOON the fruit mixture evenly over the crust and then sprinkle the reserved crumble topping evenly over the fruit.

BAKE for 40 to 45 minutes, until the topping is a nice golden brown and the fruit is bubbling.

LET the crumble cool in the pan set on a wire rack. When lukewarm, cool completely in the refrigerator before cutting into squares. Store in the refrigerator for up to 4 days or in the freezer for up to 3 months.

Tip

The coconut oil should be the texture of softened butter. If it melts to a liquid because the kitchen is too warm, refrigerate for 15 to 20 minutes until it solidifies.

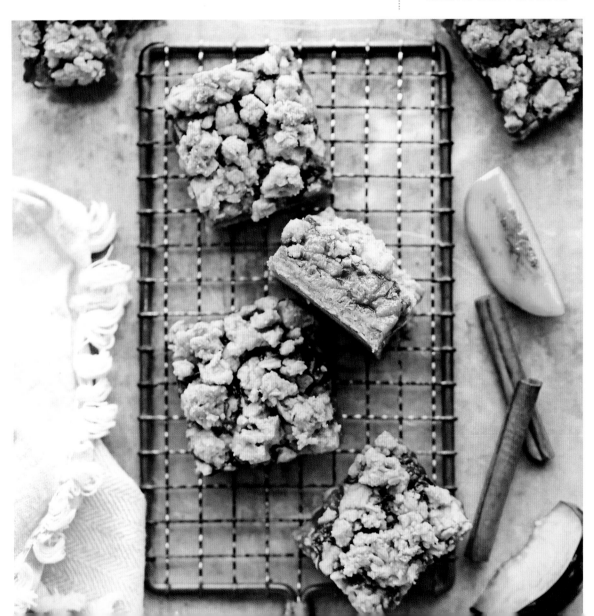

Prep time: 30 minutes
Bake time: 20 minutes
Total time: 50 minutes
Yield: 16 brookies

FOR THE COOKIE DOUGH

¼ cup (50g) refined coconut oil, softened

⅓ cup (48g) coconut sugar

½ flax egg (see Tip)

½ teaspoon pure vanilla extract

1 cup plus 2 tablespoons (108g) blanched almond flour

¼ teaspoon baking soda

¼ teaspoon kosher salt

2 ounces mini chocolate chips (about ⅓ cup)

FOR THE BROWNIE BATTER

2 ounces unsweetened chocolate, chopped (about ¼ cup)

3 tablespoons (38g) refined coconut oil

⅓ cup (113g) pure maple syrup

2 tablespoons coconut sugar

½ cup (128g) creamy natural almond butter

1½ flax eggs (see Tip)

1 teaspoon pure vanilla extract

⅓ cup (32g) blanched almond flour

⅓ cup (32g) cacao powder

½ teaspoon baking soda

½ teaspoon kosher salt

BROOKIES

PALEO • GRAIN-FREE • VEGAN • GLUTEN-FREE • DAIRY-FREE

Brownie, meet cookie. When you can't decide between a decadent, fudgy chocolate brownie and a gooey chocolate chip cookie, this is the recipe to turn to: the brookie. I've combined two of my favorite recipes—a more traditional take on the Mexican Chocolate Brownies (page 190) and my Paleo Chocolate Chip Cookies (page 149)—to create a treat that's nothing short of irresistible and perfect for when you're feeling indecisive. They're rich, so make sure you've got a glass of almond milk handy to wash them down—or even better, top with a scoop of ice cream!

FOR THE COOKIE DOUGH: In a mixing bowl, stir the coconut oil with the coconut sugar until well mixed. Add the egg and vanilla and mix again until smooth.

ADD the almond flour, baking soda, and salt to the wet ingredients. Mix until well incorporated. Fold in the mini chocolate chips.

FORM about 48 small balls of cookie dough (about 1 teaspoon each) and put on a parchment paper–lined plate. Freeze for about 15 minutes to firm up while preparing the brownie batter.

PREHEAT the oven to 350°F. Line an 8 × 8-inch baking pan with parchment paper.

FOR THE BROWNIE BATTER: Combine the unsweetened chocolate and coconut oil in a large microwave-safe bowl and microwave for 30 seconds. Stir and repeat until the chocolate and coconut oil are completely melted and smooth.

ADD the maple syrup, coconut sugar, and almond butter. Whisk well. Add the flax eggs and vanilla and whisk until combined. Add the almond flour, cacao powder, baking soda, and salt and stir well.

SPREAD the batter evenly in the lined pan. Dot the batter with the cookie dough balls, pressing them into the batter so they are partially submerged.

BAKE for 20 to 24 minutes, until a toothpick inserted in the center of the brownies comes out with a few crumbs clinging to it.

LET cool completely before cutting and serving. I like to place the pan in the fridge overnight before cutting. This makes the bars extra fudgy and much easier to cut.

STORE in an airtight container at room temperature for a few days, or in the refrigerator for up to 1 week.

Tip

To make the ½ flax egg for the cookies, whisk 1½ teaspoons ground flax seed with 1½ tablespoons water. To make the 1½ flax eggs for the brownies, whisk 1½ tablespoons ground flax seed with 5 tablespoons water. Let set for 10 minutes to give them time to gel.

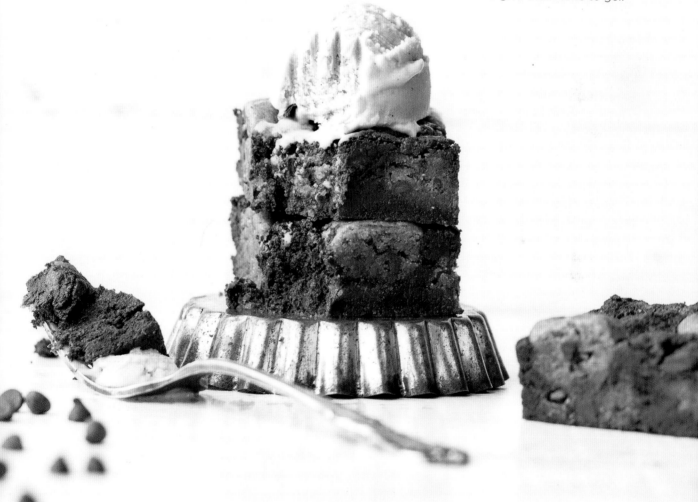

Prep time: 15 minutes
Bake time: 20 minutes
Total time: 35 minutes
Yield: 16 blondies

FOR THE BLONDIES

½ cup (128g) creamy peanut butter

¼ cup (50g) refined coconut oil, melted

¼ cup (36g) coconut sugar

5 tablespoons (106g) honey

1 flax egg (see Tip) or 1 large egg, at room temperature

1 teaspoon pure vanilla extract

1¼ cups (120g) blanched almond flour

1 teaspoon baking soda

½ teaspoon ground cinnamon

¼ teaspoon kosher salt

About 8 fresh figs, halved

FOR THE PEANUT BUTTER DRIZZLE

3 tablespoons (48g) creamy peanut butter

1 teaspoon refined coconut oil, melted

Tips

- To make a flax egg, whisk together 1 tablespoon ground flax seed with 2½ tablespoons water. Set aside for about 10 minutes to gel.
- To keep these vegan, use pure maple syrup instead of honey.

PEANUT BUTTER AND FIG BLONDIES

GRAIN-FREE • VEGAN • GLUTEN-FREE • DAIRY-FREE

In June of 2018, my older sister, Shaina, went on an eight-day silent meditation retreat. Right after she came back, she called to tell me about her experience and one of the first things she mentioned was the food. She told me about how, without distractions, she could appreciate the food so fully, tasting all the flavors and texture each bite had to offer. The meditation center had orchards where they grew their own fruit and she described eating fresh figs every morning, drizzled in peanut butter. "An interesting combo," I noted, and she requested that I create a recipe using those flavors. So here it is: peanut butter and fig blondies, a recipe we developed together just after her retreat. She was right—the fig and peanut butter flavors pair together in a beautiful way, with the richness of the peanut butter and the sweetness of the fig. The chewy blondies also feature the warm flavors of honey, vanilla, and cinnamon, which work together so wonderfully.

PREHEAT the oven to 350°F. Line an 8 × 8-inch baking pan with parchment paper and grease it lightly with coconut oil.

FOR THE BLONDIES: In a mixing bowl, stir together the peanut butter, melted coconut oil, coconut sugar, 4 tablespoons of the honey, the egg, and vanilla until smooth and well mixed. Add the almond flour, baking soda, cinnamon, and salt and stir until incorporated. Spread evenly in the prepared pan. Arrange the figs, cut sides up, on top of the batter to make a pleasing design. Press the figs slightly into the batter.

PUT the 1 remaining tablespoon honey in a small, microwave-safe bowl and microwave for about 10 seconds to liquefy. Use a pastry brush to brush the honey on top of the figs.

BAKE the blondies for 20 to 22 minutes, until golden brown. The blondies will rise a little and then collapse back onto themselves as they cool. Let them cool in the pan sitting on a wire rack. When the blondies are nearly cool, transfer to the refrigerator to cool completely.

FOR THE PEANUT BUTTER DRIZZLE: In a small bowl, whisk together the peanut butter and coconut oil. Spoon the mixture into a pastry bag, or use a zippered plastic bag by putting the mixture in the bag and snipping a corner. Drizzle the mixture over the blondies. Return the blondies to the refrigerator for 15 minutes to set the drizzle, if desired. Cut the chilled blondies into 16 squares. Refrigerate in an airtight container for up to 5 days.

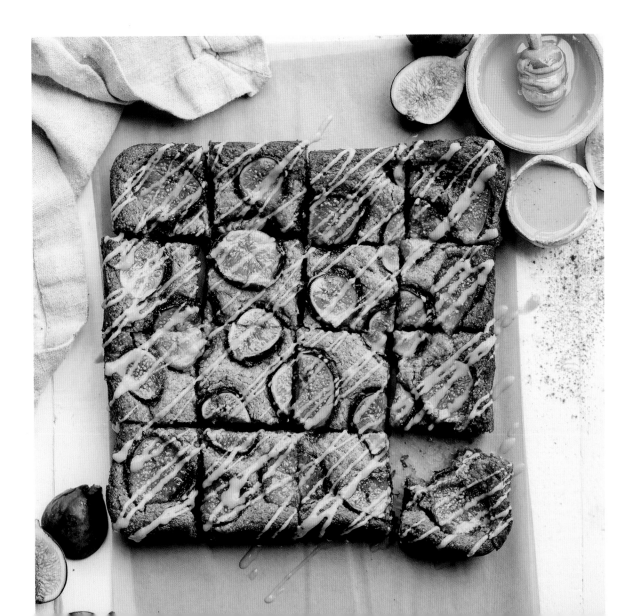

Prep time: 40 minutes
Bake time: 25 minutes
Total time: about 1 hour
Yield: 16 bars

FOR THE COCONUT MILK CARAMEL (OR SEE TIP)

1 (13.5-ounce) can full-fat coconut milk

½ cup (72g) coconut sugar

2 tablespoons coconut butter

½ teaspoon pure vanilla extract

FOR THE BARS

1 cup (96g) blanched almond flour

¼ cup (64g) coconut butter, plus more if needed, melted

½ teaspoon ground cinnamon

½ teaspoon sea salt

5 ounces bittersweet chocolate chips (about ¾ cup)

½ cup (57g) coarsely chopped walnuts

¼ cup (28g) coarsely chopped almonds

½ cup (30g) unsweetened flaked coconut

PALEO MAGIC COOKIE BARS

PALEO • GRAIN-FREE • VEGAN • GLUTEN-FREE • DAIRY-FREE

Nothing reminds me more of the holidays than magic cookie bars: layered bars traditionally made of a graham cracker crust, sweetened condensed milk, chocolate and butterscotch chips, nuts, and coconut. When I was growing up, my mom and I spent hours in the kitchen together, making pan after pan of magic cookie bars, eating butterscotch chips and coconut as we went. We cut them into small bars and stored them in Tupperware containers in the freezer in the garage. I snuck out to the garage to eat them regularly, straight from the freezer. So when both my sister and I went gluten-free, and then I went dairy-free as well, we mourned the loss of our annual magic cookie bar feast. I set out to create a version we could eat, without losing the classic flavors and textures. They may take a little longer to make because you need to make the coconut milk caramel to replace the sweetened condensed milk, but it is worth it! If you want to skip that step, you can buy sweetened condensed coconut milk. They are crunchy, chewy, and absolutely decadent—perfect for the holidays.

FOR THE COCONUT MILK CARAMEL: In a heavy saucepan, heat the coconut milk and coconut sugar over medium heat, stirring often, until the mixture begins to boil. Lower the heat and simmer until reduced by a third or half, stirring often to prevent the sugar from scorching. (If the mixture thickens and sugar begins to form on the sides or bottom of the pan, use a whisk to reincorporate it.) Simmer gently until the mixture reaches a consistency similar to thick, sweetened condensed milk or a drippy caramel sauce, about 30 minutes. Add the coconut butter and vanilla. Stir well to blend the ingredients. Remove the pan from the heat. You should end up with a little more than 1 cup of caramel-colored, sweetened coconut milk.

PREHEAT the oven to 350°F. Line an 8 × 8-inch baking pan with parchment paper and lightly grease with coconut oil.

FOR THE BARS: While the caramel simmers (be sure to continue stirring every few minutes), mix together the almond flour, coconut

CONTINUES

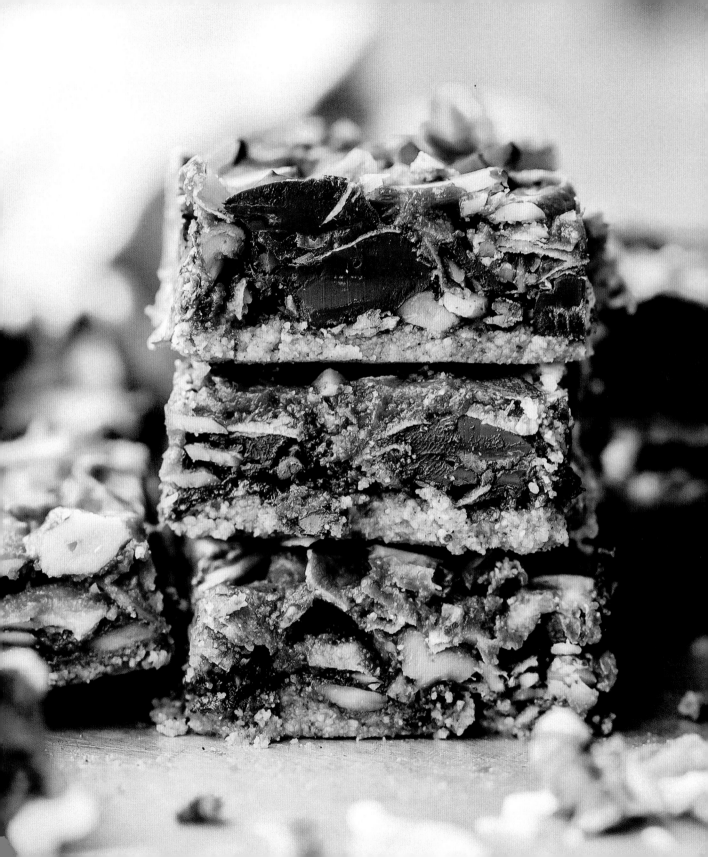

butter, cinnamon, and salt to make a dough. If the ingredients don't come together, add more coconut butter and keep stirring until it does. Sprinkle this mixture in the prepared baking pan and use your fingers or a spatula to press the mixture down in an even layer, covering the bottom.

SPRINKLE the chocolate chips, walnuts, almonds, and coconut flakes evenly over the crust. Pour the warm coconut milk caramel evenly over everything. Bake for 25 to 30 minutes, until lightly browned around the edges and bubbling.

LET the bars cool in the pan set on a wire rack. When cool, refrigerate for about 1 hour, or until completely chilled and set. Cut into 16 squares with a sharp knife and serve.

STORE in an airtight container in the refrigerator for up to a week or in the freezer for up to 3 months.

Tip

If you want to skip the initial steps of making caramel, you can buy commercially made vegan sweetened condensed milk. However, all that I've seen are made with cane sugar. If you'd like to use the store-bought version, start this recipe where it says, "Preheat the oven to 350°F."

ULTIMATE FUDGE BROWNIES

PALEO • GRAIN-FREE • GLUTEN-FREE • DAIRY-FREE

When I first started baking without gluten, dairy, and refined sugars, I wasn't entirely sure where to start. So I started with converting my favorite "regular" recipes with the new ingredients I was discovering. One of the first recipes I worked on was the favorite brownie recipe I had been making for years, which is a huge fan favorite. I subbed in almond flour for the all-purpose flour, coconut oil for the butter, and coconut sugar for the white sugar. Most everything else stayed the same. But it didn't work at first. I played around a few more times, until I landed on this version for the ultimate fudge brownies. It packs all the same fudgy, chocolatey punch as my OG favorite version. I added frosting for extra decadence, but these brownies are enough to satisfy any chocolate craving all on their own. Be sure not to add too much flour or overbake—those are the death of fudginess!

PREHEAT the oven to 350°F. Line an 8 × 8-inch baking pan with parchment paper and grease lightly with coconut oil.

FOR THE BROWNIES: In a medium bowl, whisk the almond flour with the cacao powder and salt.

PUT the chocolate and coconut oil in a large glass bowl and microwave for 30 seconds. Stir and repeat until the chocolate and coconut oil are completely melted and smooth. Add the coconut sugar. Whisk until combined. The mixture should be warm room temperature.

ADD the eggs to the chocolate mixture and whisk until combined. Add the vanilla and stir. Do not overbeat the batter at this stage or the brownies will be cakey.

SPRINKLE the flour mixture over the chocolate mixture. Using a rubber spatula, fold the flour mixture into the chocolate until combined. Fold in the chocolate chips.

SPREAD the batter into the prepared pan. Bake for 28 to 32 minutes, until a toothpick inserted in the middle of the brownies

Prep time: 10 minutes
Bake time: 28 minutes
Total time: about 40 minutes
Yield: 16 brownies

FOR THE BROWNIES
- ⅔ cup (64g) blanched almond flour
- 1 tablespoon cacao powder
- ½ teaspoon kosher salt
- 6 ounces bittersweet chocolate (see Tip), coarsely chopped (about 1 cup)
- ½ cup (100g) refined coconut oil
- ¾ cup (108g) coconut sugar
- 2 large eggs, at room temperature
- 1 teaspoon pure vanilla extract
- ½ cup mini chocolate chips

FOR THE FROSTING
- 2 ounces bittersweet chocolate, chopped (about ⅓ cup)
- 3 tablespoons (48g) creamy almond butter
- 1 tablespoon refined coconut oil
- 2 tablespoons unsweetened almond milk or other dairy-free milk
- 1 teaspoon pure vanilla extract

CONTINUES

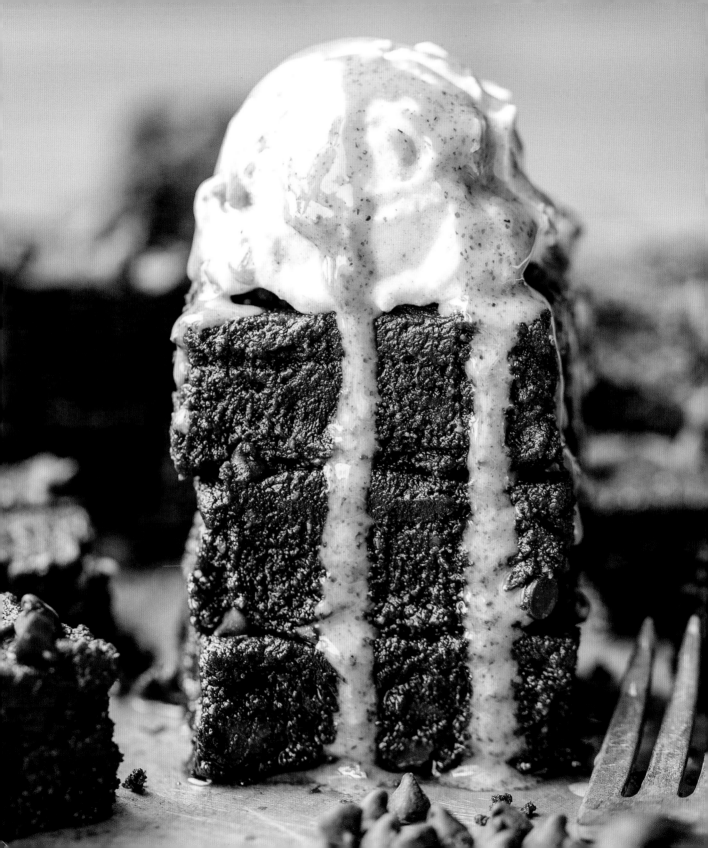

comes out with moist crumbs attached. Be careful not to overbake, or the brownies won't be fudgy! Cool the brownies completely in the pan set on a wire rack before frosting.

FOR THE FROSTING: Mix the chocolate, almond butter, and coconut oil in a small saucepan over low heat. Let the mixture melt, stirring frequently. Once melted, whisk in the almond milk and vanilla until combined. Remove from the heat. Spread the frosting on top of the cooled brownies and refrigerate until the frosting is set.

ONCE chilled, cut the brownies into 16 equal squares with a very sharp knife. The brownies will keep in an airtight container at room temperature for a few days; in the refrigerator for up to 1 week; and in the freezer for up to 3 months.

Tip

The darker the chocolate, the richer the brownie!
I use 72 percent bittersweet chocolate, which means it is
made up of 72 percent cacao products (chocolate liquor,
cocoa butter, and cacao solids), with the rest made up of sugar.
I don't recommend using chocolate with a higher percentage of
cacao unless you want these brownies super dark and bitter.
If you want a brownie that's a little sweeter than these,
60 percent cacao is a good choice.

Prep time: 15 minutes
Chill time: 1 hour
Total time: 1¼ hours
Yield: 16 bars

FOR THE CEREAL LAYER

⅔ cup (170g) cashew butter

¼ cup (64g) coconut butter, melted

2 tablespoons pure maple syrup

1 cup freeze-dried strawberries, crushed

2½ cups (78g) crispy brown rice cereal

FOR THE CHOCOLATE LAYER

3 ounces bittersweet chocolate, chopped (about 6 tablespoons)

2 tablespoons cashew butter

Freeze-dried strawberries, for garnish (optional)

CHOCOLATE-COVERED STRAWBERRY CRISPY BARS

VEGAN • NO-BAKE • GLUTEN-FREE • DAIRY-FREE

Imagine a crispy rice cereal bar, but instead of marshmallows, the cereal is coated with a sweet strawberry-flavored cashew butter. The crunchy pink base layer is topped with a thin layer of chocolate, emulating all the flavors of a chocolate-covered strawberry—a personal favorite. To keep the rice cereal from getting soggy and wet, the recipe uses freeze-dried strawberries, which pack all the flavor of ripe berries without any of the moisture. If strawberries aren't your favorite, sub in your favorite freeze-dried fruit. These are also great with Homemade White Chocolate (page 230) melted on top instead of the bittersweet chocolate.

LINE an 8 × 8-inch baking pan with parchment paper and grease lightly with coconut oil.

FOR THE CEREAL LAYER: In a medium mixing bowl, stir together the cashew butter, melted coconut butter, maple syrup, and crushed freeze-dried strawberries until combined. Using a rubber spatula or spoon, stir in the rice cereal until it is completely coated with the nut butter mixture. Press evenly into the prepared pan.

FOR THE CHOCOLATE LAYER: Put the chocolate in a microwave-safe bowl and microwave in 30-second intervals, stirring between each, until the chocolate is smooth and liquid. Whisk in the cashew butter until smooth. Spread the topping over the cereal layer. Garnish with freeze-dried strawberries, if desired.

REFRIGERATE the bars for at least 1 hour to set. Use a sharp knife to cut 16 bars. Refrigerate in an airtight container for up to 1 week.

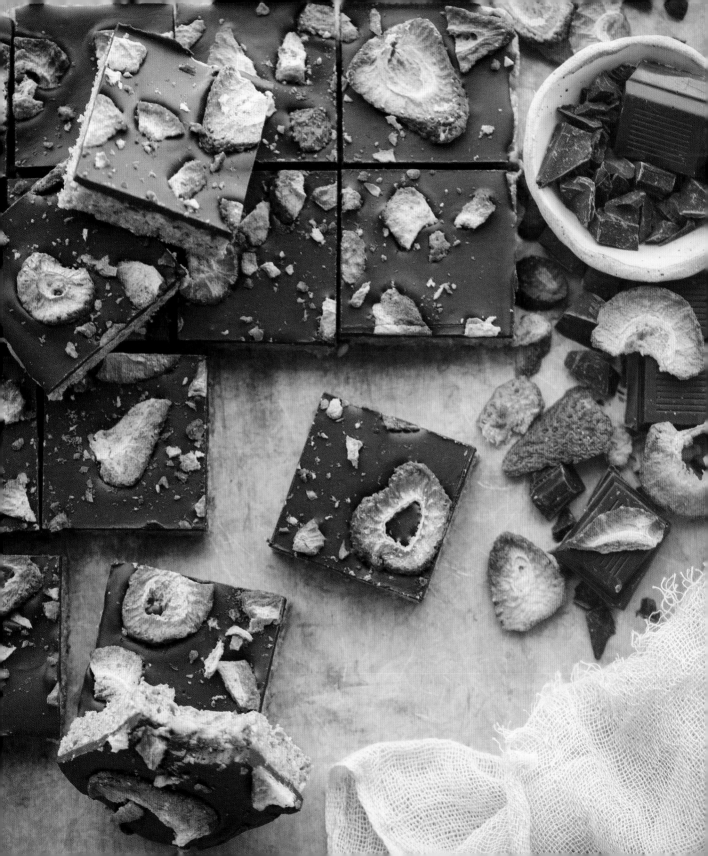

Prep time: 20 minutes
Bake time: 25 minutes
Total time: 45 minutes
Yield: 16 blondies

FOR THE BLONDIES

¼ cup (50g) refined coconut oil, melted

⅓ cup (85g) cashew or pecan butter, or any other nut butter you like

⅓ cup (48g) coconut sugar

1 flax egg (see Tip) or 1 large egg, at room temperature

1½ teaspoons pure vanilla extract

1 cup (96g) blanched almond flour

¼ teaspoon baking soda

¾ teaspoon kosher salt

FOR THE PECAN LAYER

1½ cups (170g) pecans

¼ cup (50g) refined coconut oil

¼ cup (36g) coconut sugar

2 tablespoons pure maple syrup

⅓ cup canned full-fat coconut milk

½ teaspoon kosher salt

Tip

To make a flax egg, mix 1 tablespoon ground flax seed with 2½ tablespoons water. Whisk well and then set aside at room temperature for about 10 minutes to gel.

PECAN PIE BLONDIES

PALEO • GRAIN-FREE • VEGAN • GLUTEN-FREE • DAIRY-FREE

I was always iffy on pecan pie growing up. The ones that I encountered were always less pecan and more sugary goo, of which I was not a fan (despite my sugar-loving ways). But the flavors... those I could get behind. And I always loved shortbread-crusted pecan bars, which pack in a ton of pecans without all the goo. So here I take all the goodness of the pecan pie and pile it on top of a buttery, chewy blondie—similar to a pecan pie bar but with a decadent blondie instead of the shortbread. The only "goo" is a sticky, caramel-like layer that holds the pecans together, and it creates an incredible dessert that I'd be happy to serve on the holidays.

PREHEAT the oven to 350°F. Line an 8 × 8-inch baking pan with parchment paper and grease with coconut oil.

FOR THE BLONDIES: Whisk together the melted coconut oil and nut butter. Add the coconut sugar, egg, and vanilla and whisk to combine. Add the almond flour, baking soda, and salt and stir until combined. Pour the batter into the prepared pan and smooth it lightly with a spatula or offset knife. The layer will be quite thin.

FOR THE PECAN LAYER: Spread the pecans in a single layer in a dry skillet. Toast over medium heat, stirring frequently, until the nuts are aromatic and lightly browned, 6 to 7 minutes. Slide the toasted nuts from the pan onto a plate and let them cool. When cool enough to handle, roughly chop.

MELT the coconut oil in a saucepan over medium heat. Once melted, whisk in the coconut sugar and maple syrup and continue whisking until the sugar is dissolved. Bring to a boil, stirring occasionally. Once the mixture reaches a boil, cook for 1 minute. Remove from the heat and then stir in the coconut milk and salt. Add the pecans, stir well, and pour the mixture evenly over the blondie layer.

BAKE for 25 to 30 minutes, until the bars are just set around the edges but still bubbling.

SET the pan on a wire rack and let the blondies cool completely. Slice the cooled blondies into 16 squares for serving. I like to refrigerate the cooled bars for a few hours to make them easier to cut.

THE blondies can be refrigerated in an airtight container for up to 1 week, or frozen for up to 3 months.

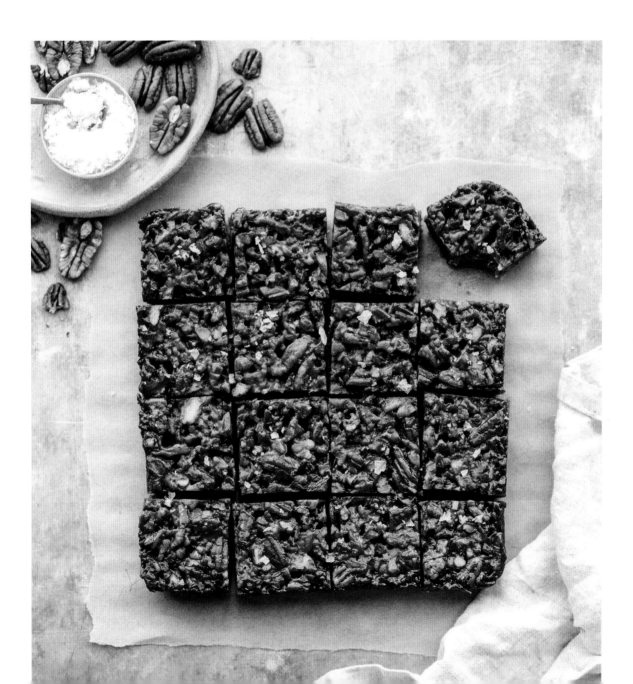

Prep time: 20 minutes

Bake time: 15 minutes

Chill time: 1 hour

Total time: about 1½ hours

Yield: 16 bars

FOR THE SHORTBREAD CRUST

3 tablespoons (63g) pure maple syrup

⅓ cup (67g) refined coconut oil, slightly softened (see Tip)

⅔ cup (86g) coconut flour

¼ teaspoon kosher salt

FOR THE CARAMEL COCONUT FILLING

¾ cup (85g) unsweetened shredded coconut

½ cup (128g) creamy almond butter

⅓ cup (113g) pure maple syrup

⅓ cup (85g) coconut butter or (66g) refined coconut oil

1 teaspoon pure vanilla extract

¼ teaspoon kosher salt

4½ ounces bittersweet chocolate, chopped (about ¾ cup)

Tip

The coconut oil should be the texture of softened butter. If it melts to a liquid because the kitchen is too warm, refrigerate for 15 to 20 minutes until it solidifies.

CHOCOLATE-DRIZZLED COCONUT BARS

PALEO • GRAIN-FREE • VEGAN • GLUTEN-FREE • DAIRY-FREE

Calling all coconut fans! If your favorite Girl Scout cookie growing up was a Samoa (also called Caramel deLite), you've found your way to the right recipe. With a crunchy shortbread crust, a coconut-filled, caramel-like topping, and a dunk and drizzle of chocolate, these re-create all those nostalgic flavors, but in a way that's much easier to make than cut-out cookies. With only nine ingredients, they come together quickly, and will probably get devoured just as quickly. If they make it that long, they're also perfect for freezing to have on hand whenever you need a sweet treat.

PREHEAT the oven to 350°F. Line an 8 × 8-inch baking pan with parchment paper and grease with coconut oil. Line a baking sheet with parchment paper.

FOR THE CRUST: In a mixing bowl, stir the maple syrup and coconut oil until well mixed. Add the coconut flour and salt and stir until the dough comes together. Make sure to press out any clumps of coconut oil. Use your hands to bring the dough fully together so that it's completely smooth. You can also mix it in a stand mixer fitted with the paddle attachment.

PRESS the dough into the prepared pan, covering the bottom in a flat layer. Bake the crust for 15 to 17 minutes, until golden brown around the edges. Let cool completely.

FOR THE FILLING: Spread the shredded coconut in a large skillet so that it makes a single layer. Set over medium heat and toast for 3 to 4 minutes, stirring often to ensure even browning, until the coconut begins to brown. Remove the skillet from the heat and let the coconut finish toasting in the hot pan, about 10 minutes, stirring every few minutes. Shake the toasted coconut from the skillet and let it cool completely.

IN a small saucepan, heat the almond butter, maple syrup, coconut butter, vanilla, and salt over medium heat until all the ingredients are melted and thoroughly combined. Alternatively, you can heat the ingredients in the microwave for 45 seconds, or until melted and smooth. Add the toasted coconut and stir to mix well. Pour the mixture over the crust. Refrigerate until set, about 1 hour.

CUT the coconut bars into 16 square bars. Put ½ cup of the chopped chocolate in a small microwave-safe bowl and microwave for about 30 seconds. Stir the chocolate and if it's not smooth and liquefied, microwave for 30 seconds longer.

DIP the bottom of each bar into the melted chocolate, scrape off the excess chocolate on the side of the bowl, and put the bars on the lined baking sheet to set.

MELT the remaining ¼ cup chocolate in the microwave and transfer to a small piping bag or zippered plastic bag with the corner snipped off. Drizzle the chocolate over the bars.

STORE any leftovers tightly sealed in the refrigerator for up to 1 week, or in the freezer for up to 3 months. These are delicious frozen!

Prep time: 20 minutes
Bake time: 35 minutes
Total time: about 1 hour
Yield: 16 bars

FOR THE RHUBARB
6 to 8 fresh rhubarb stalks, cut into 7-inch-long pieces (see Tips)

2 tablespoons honey or pure maple syrup

1 tablespoon grated orange zest

1 tablespoon orange juice

¼ teaspoon vanilla bean powder

FOR THE CRUST
⅓ cup (113g) pure maple syrup

2 tablespoons (32g) almond butter

½ cup (100g) refined coconut oil, softened

¾ cup (72g) blanched almond flour

¾ cup (96g) coconut flour

⅓ cup (37g) shelled raw pistachios, finely chopped

FOR THE PISTACHIO FRANGIPANE
¾ cup (84g) shelled raw pistachios

1 tablespoon tapioca flour

⅓ cup (48g) coconut sugar

¼ teaspoon kosher salt

5 tablespoons (63g) refined coconut oil, softened

1 flax egg (see Tips) or 1 large egg, at room temperature

1 teaspoon pure vanilla extract

RHUBARB-PISTACHIO FRANGIPANE BARS
PALEO • GRAIN-FREE • VEGAN • GLUTEN-FREE • DAIRY-FREE

Have you had frangipane before? It's a sweet paste, typically made with almonds that have been pureed with butter, sugar, and eggs, and it's used in pastries like fruit tarts. For these bars, we make a frangipane filling, but instead of almonds we use nutrient-dense pistachios and switch out the butter, sugar, and eggs for coconut oil, coconut sugar, and a flax egg. The pistachio frangipane is spread onto a pistachio-studded shortbread crust and topped with stalks of red rhubarb that have been macerated in honey, vanilla, and orange zest. The rich sweetness of the pistachio crust and pistachio frangipane filling make a perfect foil for the tartness of the rhubarb. If rhubarb isn't in season, try using halved strawberries.

FOR THE RHUBARB: Put the rhubarb in a bowl or baking dish and add the honey, orange zest and juice, and vanilla. Toss to coat the rhubarb and set aside to macerate at room temperature while you prepare the crust and frangipane.

FOR THE CRUST: Line a 9 × 9-inch baking pan or 9-inch tart pan with parchment paper. Grease lightly with coconut oil.

IN a mixing bowl, combine the maple syrup, almond butter, and coconut oil and stir until combined. Fold in the almond flour, coconut flour, and chopped pistachios. Stir until the dry ingredients are completely moistened. Press the crust evenly into the prepared pan and refrigerate.

FOR THE FRANGIPANE: Preheat the oven to 350°F.

IN the bowl of a food processor fitted with the metal blade or high-powered blender (I use a Vitamix), grind the pistachios, tapioca flour, coconut sugar, and salt to a powder, or as fine as you can make it. Add the coconut oil and process until it is no longer visible. Add the egg and vanilla, blending until completely incorporated and a smooth paste forms. Spread the filling evenly over the crust.

CONTINUES

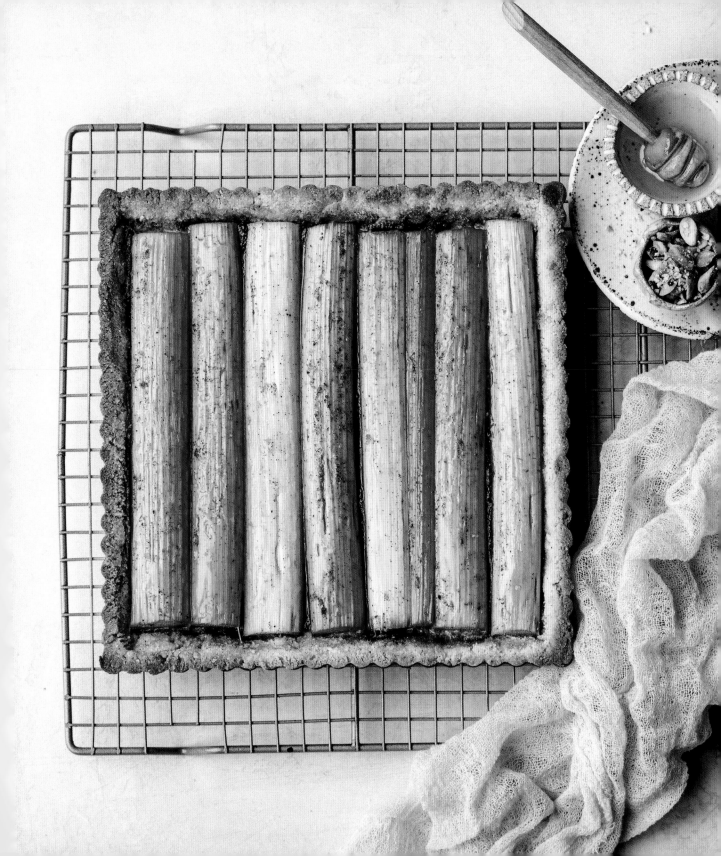

Tips

- If you prefer, cut the rhubarb into smaller lengths to make them a little easier to eat.
- To make a flax egg, whisk 1 tablespoon ground flax seed with 2½ tablespoons water. Set aside for about 10 minutes to give the mixture time to gel.

LIFT the rhubarb from the dish, letting any excess liquid drip back into the dish. Arrange them over the pistachio paste in a pleasing pattern.

BAKE for 35 to 40 minutes, until the crust is golden brown and a skewer inserted into the center comes out clean.

LET the bars cool completely before cutting into squares. Refrigerate, well wrapped, for 3 to 4 days, or freeze for a few months.

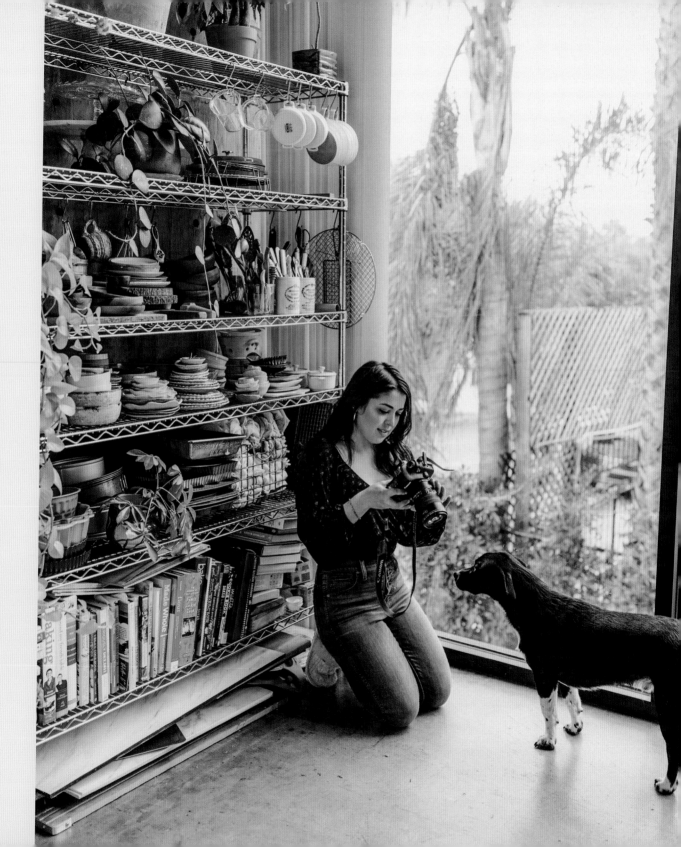

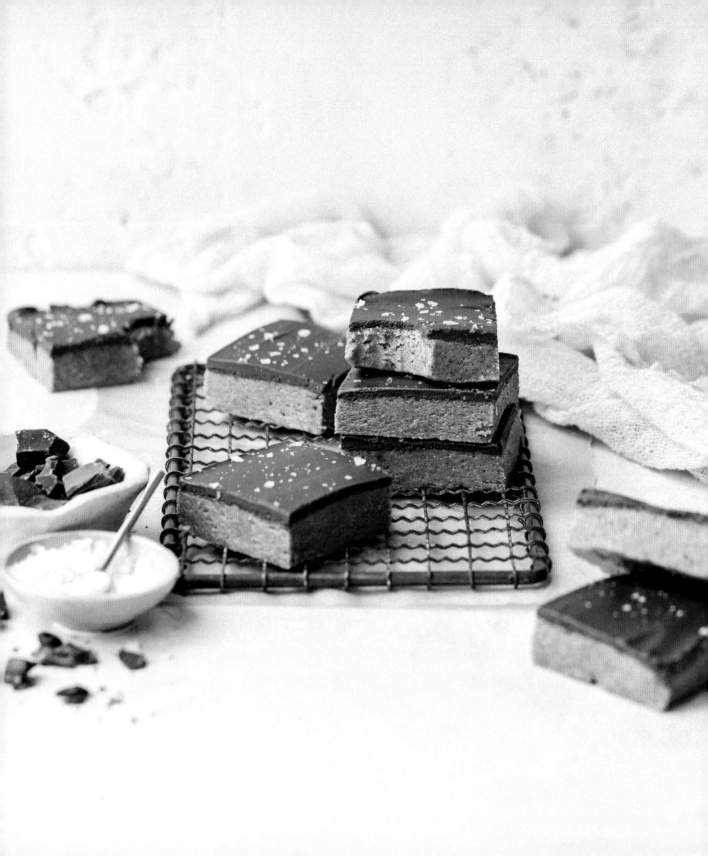

NO-BAKE CHOCOLATE–ALMOND BUTTER BARS

PALEO • GRAIN-FREE • VEGAN • NO-BAKE • GLUTEN-FREE • DAIRY-FREE

These bars are for the people who see a chocolate–nut butter cup and want to up the nut butter ratio by a lot—I'm one of those people. This recipe uses a ton of almond butter to create a thick and creamy nut butter base, with some maple syrup stirred in for sweetness and coconut oil and coconut flour to help firm up the nut butter. Then chocolate is mixed with almond butter, which helps keep the chocolate fudgier and not as brittle, for the topping. The result is an easy-to-make bar that melts in your mouth and is even easier to eat. Try out any of your favorite nut butters to switch up the flavor.

LINE an 8 × 8-inch baking pan with parchment paper and grease lightly with coconut oil.

FOR THE BASE: In a mixing bowl, stir together the almond butter, coconut oil, maple syrup, coconut flour, and salt. Press evenly into the prepared pan and refrigerate.

FOR THE CHOCOLATE TOPPING: Put the chocolate and almond butter in a microwave-safe bowl. Microwave in 30-second intervals, stirring between each, until the chocolate mixture is melted and smooth, 1 to 1½ minutes. Pour the chocolate over the almond butter base and spread it to cover the top of the base. Sprinkle with the sea salt.

REFRIGERATE for at least 2 hours. Use a sharp knife to cut the bars into 16 servings. Refrigerate the bars, tightly wrapped, for up to 2 weeks.

Prep time: 10 minutes
Chill time: 2 hours
Total time: about 2¼ hours
Yield: 16 bars

FOR THE BASE
1½ cups (384g) creamy almond butter

⅓ cup (67g) refined coconut oil, melted

¼ cup (85g) pure maple syrup

¼ cup (32g) coconut flour

¼ teaspoon kosher salt (skip if the nut butter is salted)

FOR THE CHOCOLATE TOPPING
4 ounces bittersweet chocolate, finely chopped (about ⅔ cup)

2 tablespoons creamy almond butter

Flaky sea salt, for sprinkling

Prep time: 30 minutes

Bake time: 10 minutes

Total time: 40 minutes plus chilling and setting

Yield: 16 bars

FOR THE CHOCOLATE CRUST

¾ cup (96g) coconut flour

¼ cup (24g) cacao powder

½ teaspoon kosher salt

⅓ cup (113g) pure maple syrup

½ cup (100g) refined coconut oil, softened (see Tip)

FOR THE PEPPERMINT FILLING

¾ cup (192g) coconut butter, melted

¼ cup (50g) refined coconut oil, melted

2 tablespoons pure maple syrup

1 teaspoon peppermint extract

½ teaspoon pure vanilla extract

FOR THE CHOCOLATE TOPPING

¼ cup (50g) refined coconut oil, melted

¼ cup (24g) cacao powder

3 tablespoons (63g) pure maple syrup

½ teaspoon peppermint extract

Tip

The coconut oil should be the texture of softened butter. If it melts to a liquid, refrigerate for 15 to 20 minutes until it solidifies.

CHOCOLATE PEPPERMINT BARS

PALEO • GRAIN-FREE • VEGAN • GLUTEN-FREE • DAIRY-FREE

With a crisp chocolate shortbread crust, a creamy peppermint filling, and a layer of homemade chocolate on top, these bars are a chocolate-peppermint lover's dream. The homemade chocolate is made with a simple combination of coconut oil, cacao powder, pure maple syrup, and a little peppermint extract. There are a lot of coconut products in this recipe, but I wouldn't say the flavor is coconutty; the peppermint and chocolate flavors overshadow any coconut taste. They're also nut-free, since they use coconut flour in the crust and coconut butter in the filling.

PREHEAT the oven to 350°F. Line an 8 × 8-inch baking pan with parchment paper, then grease it lightly with coconut oil.

FOR THE CRUST: Whisk the coconut flour with the cacao powder and salt. In a separate bowl, whisk the maple syrup and coconut oil until smooth. Add the dry ingredients to the wet ingredients and stir until fully mixed and a smooth dough forms.

PRESS the dough into the prepared pan. Dock the dough (punch the dough all over with a fork to make small indentations) to prevent it from puffing up during baking. Bake for 10 to 12 minutes, until the dough looks dry and baked through. Let the crust cool completely in the pan set on a wire cooling rack.

FOR THE FILLING: In a medium bowl, combine the melted coconut butter, coconut oil, maple syrup, peppermint extract, and vanilla extract. Whisk until smooth and then pour over the cooled crust. Spread the filling into a flat, even layer. Refrigerate for at least 1 hour or until the filling hardens.

FOR THE TOPPING: While the coconut layer hardens, make the chocolate topping. In a bowl, whisk together the melted coconut oil, cacao powder, maple syrup, and peppermint extract. Pour this over the hardened coconut layer, spreading it evenly.

REFRIGERATE the bars for about 30 minutes to set. When set, cut into 16 squares. Refrigerate in an airtight container for 5 to 6 days.

STRAWBERRY SHORTCAKE BARS

PALEO • GRAIN-FREE • VEGAN • NO-BAKE • GLUTEN-FREE • DAIRY-FREE

This is one of the first cashew-based desserts I ever made (clearly by the number of cashew-centric recipes in this book, I'm a big fan now). It helped me fall in love with the creamy texture and luxurious flavors that can be created with raw cashews, without any baking necessary. The flavors here closely mimic the mouthwatering flavors of the other Strawberry Shortcakes in this book (page 107), but as a no-baking-necessary, refreshing bar dessert. On a hot summer day, there's nothing better than grabbing one out of the freezer to help cool you down!

BEFORE you begin, soak the cashews for the filling. Put the 2 cups cashews in a large bowl and add enough water to cover by 1 or 2 inches. I prefer to use filtered water but tap water is also fine. Let the cashews soak for at least 4 hours on the countertop. If soaking longer, refrigerate for up to 12 hours. If you don't have time for the longer soak, cover the cashews with boiling water and let them soak for 1 hour. This speeds up the process, although the nuts won't be as creamy as after a longer soak. Drain and rinse the cashews before using.

LINE an 8 × 8-inch baking pan with parchment paper and grease well with coconut oil.

FOR THE CRUST: In the bowl of a food processor fitted with the metal blade or a high-powered blender (I use a Vitamix but most powerful blenders should do the job), mix the ¾ cup raw cashews (not the soaked nuts) with the almond flour, pitted dates, coconut oil, and salt and pulse until the ingredients come together in a sort of sticky dough. Don't overprocess or the dough will turn into nut butter! Press the date dough evenly along the bottom of the prepared pan.

FOR THE FILLING: In the same food processor or high-powered blender, combine the drained cashews, coconut milk, coconut oil, maple syrup, lemon juice, and vanilla and blend until silky smooth

CONTINUES

Prep time: 20 minutes
Chill time: 3 hours
Total time: about 3¼ hours
Yield: 16 bars

2 cups (240g) raw cashews

FOR THE CRUST
¾ cup (90g) raw cashews
¼ cup (24g) blanched almond flour
4 Medjool dates, pitted
2 tablespoons refined coconut oil
¼ teaspoon kosher salt

FOR THE FILLING
½ cup canned full-fat coconut milk
¼ cup (50g) refined coconut oil, melted and cooled
⅓ cup (113g) pure maple syrup
2 tablespoons fresh lemon juice
1 tablespoon pure vanilla extract, or ¾ teaspoon vanilla bean powder
2 cups hulled and halved fresh or frozen strawberries

and creamy, about 2 minutes. Scrape down the sides of the bowl or blender as necessary. You may need to add more coconut milk or lemon juice to get the filling to blend smoothly, especially if your blender isn't super high powered. Once it's smooth, taste the filling and adjust the sweetness and tartness levels, if desired.

POUR the filling into the prepared pan over the crust. Smooth the top and tap the pan hard against the counter a few times to release any air bubbles. Press the strawberry halves into the bars as desired. I like putting them cut side up.

REFRIGERATE or freeze the shortcake bars for at least 3 to 6 hours to give it time to firm up. It should be completely firm before cutting. I recommend running the knife under hot water to warm it up and drying it before cutting the bars with the still-hot knife. If frozen, let the bars thaw at room temperature for 10 to 15 minutes before serving. Well-wrapped, the bars can be frozen for up to 3 months.

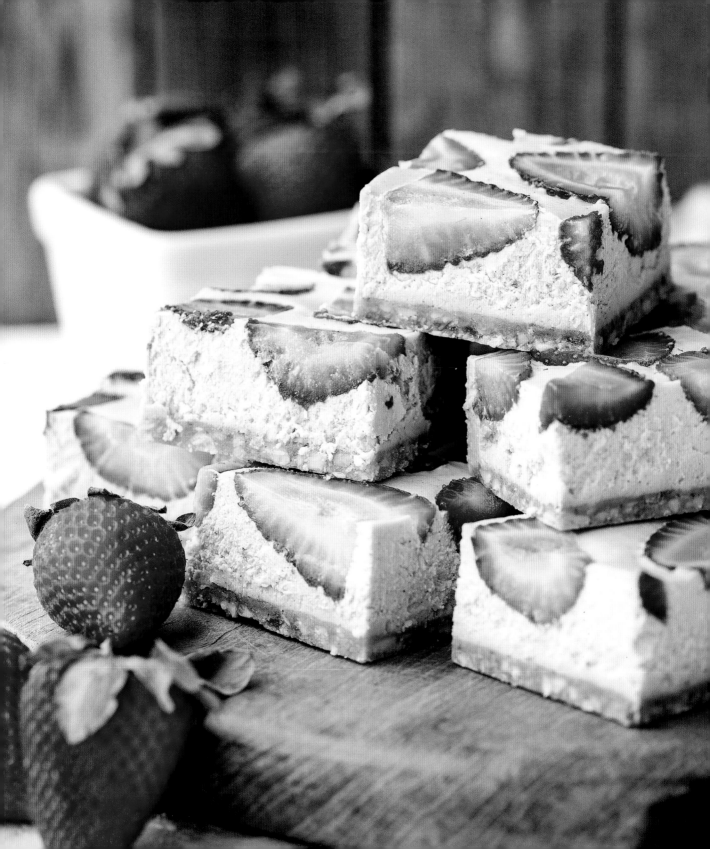

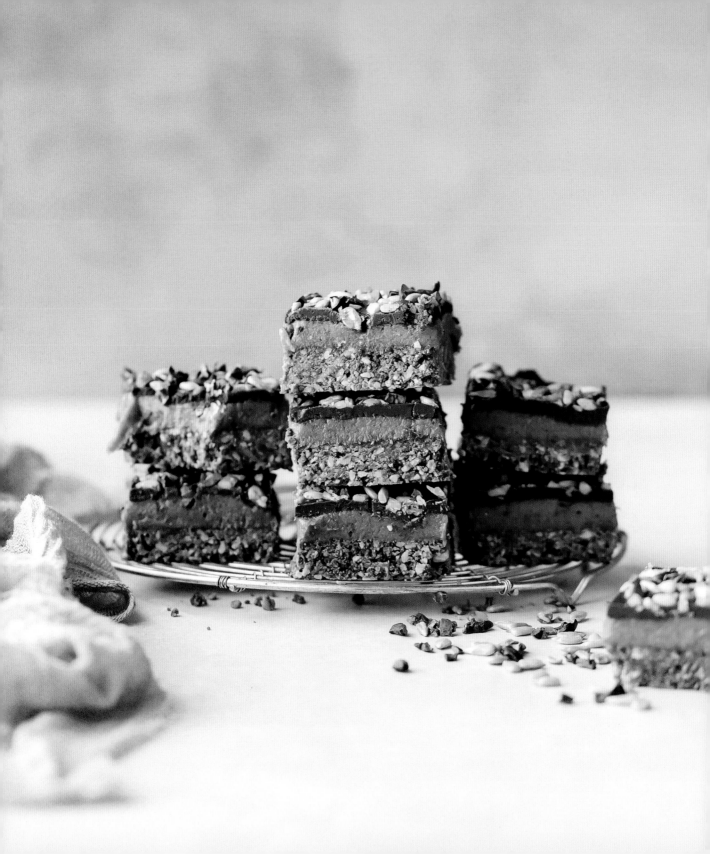

SUNFLOWER SEED AND DATE-CARAMEL BARS

PALEO • GRAIN-FREE • VEGAN • NO-BAKE • NUT-FREE • GLUTEN-FREE • DAIRY-FREE

Imagine sinking your teeth into a thick, chocolatey base, chewy and crunchy from shredded coconut and sunflower seeds, that is topped with a lusciously smooth, sticky, and naturally sweet date caramel. Layered on top is a rich chocolate ganache, with crunch from a smattering of sunflower seeds and cacao nibs. The bitterness of the cacao balanced with the sweetness of the dates creates a nut-free bar that dreams are made of.

LINE an 8 × 8-inch baking pan with parchment paper and lightly grease with coconut oil.

FOR THE CRUST: In the bowl of a food processor fitted with the metal blade or a high-powered blender (I use a Vitamix), combine all the crust ingredients. Pulse until the mixture comes together as a dough when pressed between your fingers. Transfer to the prepared pan and press evenly over the bottom of the pan.

FOR THE DATE CARAMEL: In the bowl of a food processor fitted with the metal blade or a high-powered blender (I use a Vitamix), combine all of the date-caramel ingredients and blend until perfectly smooth, scraping down the sides of the bowl or blender as necessary. Spoon over the prepared crust and smooth the top with a rubber spatula.

FOR THE TOPPING: Combine the chocolate and coconut milk in a microwave-safe bowl. Microwave for 30 seconds and then stir. If not fully melted, microwave for 15 to 30 seconds longer. Repeat as needed.

ONCE melted, pour the chocolate over the date-caramel layer and spread evenly. Top with the sunflower seeds, cacao nibs, and sea salt.

REFRIGERATE for at least 1 hour to firm the chocolate layer before cutting into 16 squares with a sharp knife.

STORE in an airtight container in the refrigerator for up to 1 week.

Prep time: 20 minutes
Chill time: 1 hour
Total time: 1 hour 20 minutes
Yield: 16 bars

FOR THE CRUST
1 cup (140g) sunflower seeds
½ cup (57g) shredded coconut
5 Medjool dates, pitted
¼ cup (64g) coconut butter, melted
3 tablespoons (18g) cacao powder
3 tablespoons (48g) sunflower seed butter

FOR THE DATE-CARAMEL LAYER
1½ cups Medjool dates, pitted (17 or 18 dates)
¼ cup full-fat coconut milk
2 tablespoons sunflower seed butter
2 tablespoons coconut butter, melted
1 teaspoon pure vanilla extract
Pinch of kosher salt

FOR THE CHOCOLATE TOPPING
4 ounces bittersweet chocolate, chopped or in chips (about ⅔ cup)
3 tablespoons canned full-fat coconut milk
1 tablespoon sunflower seeds
1 tablespoon cacao nibs
Flaky sea salt

Prep time: 20 minutes

Bake time: 45 minutes

Total time: about 1 hour

Yield: 16 bars

FOR THE CRUST

1¼ cups (120g) blanched almond flour

2 tablespoons tapioca flour

2 tablespoons refined coconut oil, melted

2 tablespoons pure maple syrup

⅛ teaspoon kosher salt

FOR THE TOPPING

1 cup (147g) raw almonds

½ cup (72g) coconut sugar

1 tablespoon tapioca flour

¼ teaspoon kosher salt

6 tablespoons (75g) refined coconut oil, softened (see Tip)

1 large egg or flax egg, at room temperature

¼ teaspoon vanilla bean powder or 1 teaspoon pure vanilla extract

¼ teaspoon almond extract

2 cups fresh blackberries (about ¾ pint), lightly mashed with a fork

Tip

The coconut oil should be the texture of softened butter. If it melts to a liquid because the kitchen is too warm, refrigerate for 15 to 20 minutes until it solidifies.

BLACKBERRY BLISS FRANGIPANE BARS

PALEO • GRAIN-FREE • VEGAN • GLUTEN-FREE • DAIRY-FREE

I've tended to overlook blackberries in my kitchen in favor of the other, more colorful berries. But these bars beg for your attention with their vibrant color and sweet flavor. The almond frangipane, which is a sweet and nutty paste, is scented with vanilla bean powder and almond extract. It balances the tart flavors from the blackberries so wonderfully. When mashed up, the blackberries form a jammy layer on top of the decadent frangipane filling, which is so well complemented by the crispy crust. I prefer the frangipane bars straight from the fridge—when they're chilled, they have an almost fudgy texture that's irresistible.

PREHEAT the oven to 350°F. Line an 8 × 8-inch baking pan with parchment paper. Grease the paper with coconut oil.

FOR THE CRUST: In a mixing bowl, stir together the almond flour, tapioca flour, coconut oil, maple syrup, and salt until fully combined. Press the crust evenly into the bottom of the pan.

FOR THE TOPPING: In the bowl of a processor fitted with the metal blade or a high-powered blender (I use a Vitamix), grind the almonds, coconut sugar, tapioca flour, and salt to a powder. Add the coconut oil and process until it's completely blended. Add the egg, vanilla, and almond extract and blend to a smooth paste. Spread the filling evenly over the almond crust. Spread the mashed blackberries evenly over the almond paste.

BAKE for 45 to 60 minutes (the time will depend on the juiciness of the blackberries). The bars are done when the filling does not jiggle if you shake the pan, and a toothpick inserted into the center comes out clean (or with just a bit of blackberry juice on it).

LET the bars cool in the pan for 20 minutes before refrigerating them to cool completely. When cool, cut into 16 squares. Refrigerate the bars in an airtight container for up to 1 week, or wrap tightly and place in an airtight container to freeze for up to 3 months.

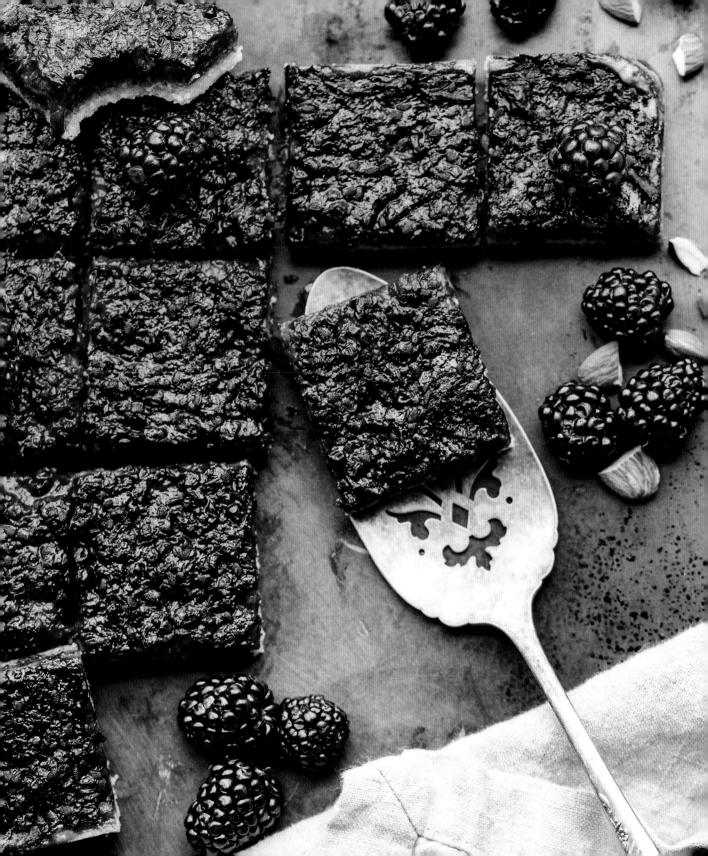

CHAPTER SIX

Candy and Confections

A FEW TIPS AND TRICKS FOR SUCCESS:
Most of these confections are best stored in the refrigerator because they get too soft if left at room temperature for too long, so please note the storage instructions for each recipe.

Feel free to switch around nut butters to create your own unique flavors! For example, you can use any type or flavor of nut butter for the Chocolate–Peanut Butter Cups.

Many of these recipes call for cacao butter. If you can't get your hands on it, refined coconut oil can be used, but it will make the melting temperature lower and the taste will be a little bit different.

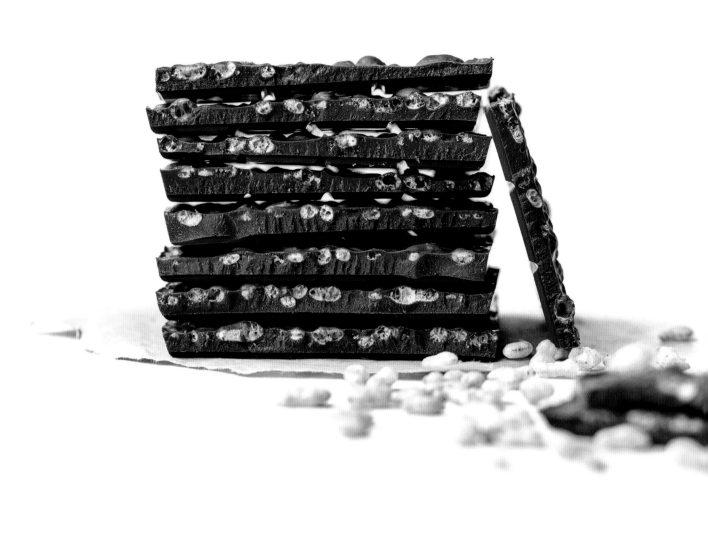

CRUNCHY BARS

VEGAN • NUT-FREE • NO-BAKE • GLUTEN-FREE • DAIRY-FREE

One way to make chocolate even more delicious? Add airy, puffy rice cereal! The traditional Crunch bar that we all grew up with has a too-long ingredients list and is filled with gluten, refined sugars, and three different kinds of dairy. Thankfully, it's a treat that's undoubtedly easy to re-create: just five wholesome ingredients and 5 minutes of prep. They're a delicious dessert on their own, or can be chopped up to use in any treats that call for chocolate chunks!

Prep time: 5 minutes
Chill time: 1 hour
Total time: about 1 hour
Yield: 2 bars or 6 crunchy mounds

2 ounces cacao butter, chopped finely if not already in chips (about ⅓ cup)

2 tablespoons (42g) pure maple syrup

⅓ cup (28g) cocoa powder

Pinch of kosher salt

¼ cup (9g) crispy brown rice cereal

COMBINE the cacao butter and maple syrup in a microwave-safe liquid measuring cup. Microwave in 20-second intervals to melt the ingredients. Stir the ingredients between each interval until completely melted, about 1 minute.

STIR in the cocoa powder and salt until completely smooth and no clumps remain. Slowly stir in the rice cereal so that it's completely coated.

SCRAPE the mixture into a chocolate bar mold (mine makes two chocolate bars) or a chocolate truffle mold. You could also use cupcake liners to hold five or six truffle-sized mounds. Refrigerate until hardened, about 1 hour.

RELEASE the bars from the molds if using, or remove them from the cupcake liners and serve. To store, put the candies in a zippered plastic bag or an airtight container, or wrap the bars in plastic wrap. Store at cool room temperature or in the refrigerator for up to 1 month.

Prep time: 10 minutes
Total time: 10 minutes
Yield: 16 bites

- ½ cup (128g) cashew butter or another creamy nut or seed butter
- ¼ cup (85g) pure maple syrup
- 1 cup (96g) blanched almond flour
- ¼ cup (24g) cacao powder
- ¼ to ½ teaspoon kosher salt
- ½ teaspoon pure vanilla extract
- 1½ ounces mini chocolate chips (about ¼ cup)
- Flaky sea salt, to garnish (optional)

SALTED BROWNIE ENERGY BITES

PALEO • GRAIN-FREE • VEGAN • NO-BAKE • GLUTEN-FREE • DAIRY-FREE

Sometimes you want a snack that will give you an energetic boost . . . but you also want it to taste like dessert. That's where these energy bites come in. They're loaded with healthy fats from cashew butter and have almond flour to fuel you and keep you full, with cacao powder, vanilla, and chocolate chips mixed in to make them taste like dessert. Don't forget a sprinkle of flaky sea salt on top to garnish! It helps cut through the richness of the chocolate and makes the bites even more irresistible.

IN a mixing bowl, stir together the cashew butter and maple syrup. Stir in the almond flour, cacao powder, ¼ teaspoon kosher salt, the vanilla, and chocolate chips. Taste the mixture and add more salt if you prefer these saltier (as I do!).

ROLL the dough into 16 balls, 1 heaping tablespoon dough each. Sprinkle with a little flaky sea salt, if desired (I recommend you do). You might need to press the salt into the dough to help it stick.

SERVE the bites now or refrigerate them for at least 45 minutes to give them time to firm up and the flavors to develop. Store in an airtight container in the refrigerator for up to 2 weeks.

Variation

PEPPERMINT BROWNIE BITES: Substitute peppermint extract for the vanilla extract and leave off the salt garnish.

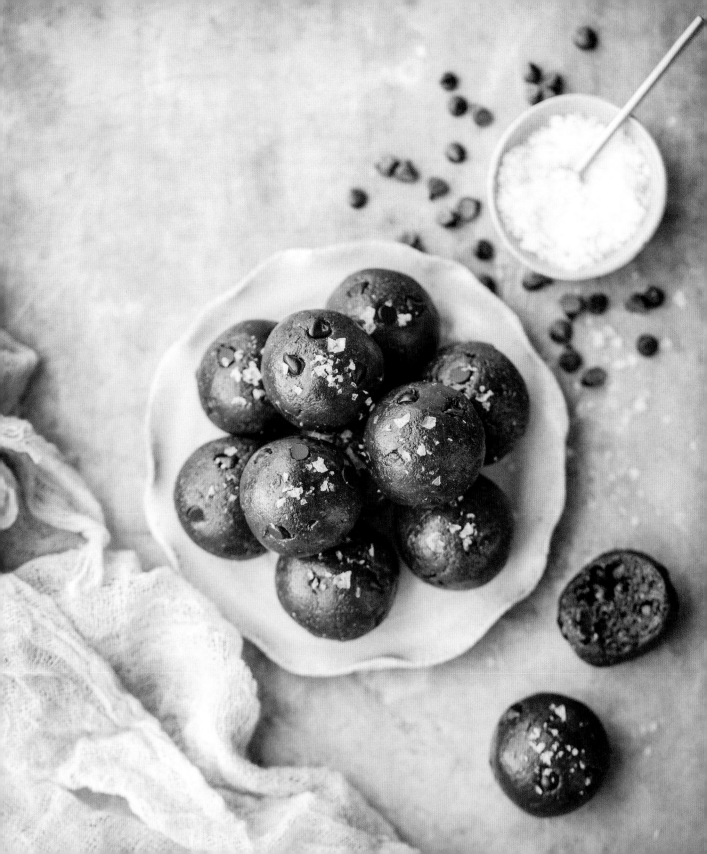

Prep time: 5 minutes

Chill time: 1 hour

Total time: about 1 hour

Yield: 2 to 3 chocolate bars, depending on size (about 2 cups chopped chocolate chunks)

....

3 ounces pure cacao butter, chopped (about ⅓ cup)

¼ cup (85g) pure maple syrup

½ cup (128g) raw cashew butter

2 tablespoons coconut milk powder (optional but recommended, if you can find it)

1 teaspoon pure vanilla extract

Pinch of salt (optional)

HOMEMADE WHITE CHOCOLATE

PALEO • GRAIN-FREE • VEGAN • NO-BAKE • GLUTEN-FREE • DAIRY-FREE

Although I started testing this recipe when I first started working on this cookbook, it was one of the last recipes to be finished. I almost gave up because I didn't just want a homemade dairy-free, refined sugar-free white chocolate. I wanted one that you can *bake* with, and let's just say that didn't happen easily. Most of the initial tests melted into oblivion once they were baked into a cookie—without milk to stabilize, the cacao butter acted like oil. I found that cashew butter and coconut milk powder can provide the creaminess and stability that normally comes from milk, while maple syrup provides the sweetness. You can chop this white chocolate up and use it in cookies (like the White Chocolate–Macadamia Nut Cookies on page 153), or use it as a white chocolate coating when it's still melted. Something to note: Because of the maple syrup, this white chocolate is more cream-colored than pure white!

....

COMBINE the cacao butter and maple syrup in a heatproof, microwave-safe bowl or liquid measuring cup. Microwave in 30-second intervals until the cacao butter melts, about 1 minute.

ADD the cashew butter, coconut milk powder if using, vanilla, and salt if using. Mix until smooth.

TRANSFER to a liquid measuring cup with a pouring spout, then pour into a chocolate bar mold or any other silicone mold (any flexible container will do). Refrigerate for about 1 hour, or until solid.

REMOVE the solid pieces of white chocolate from the molds and store, tightly wrapped in plastic or in an airtight container, in the refrigerator for 3 or 4 months.

ALTERNATIVELY, if you plan to use the white chocolate as a coating, as soon as it's mixed, dip the items of your choice (such as pretzels, strawberries, etc.) into the melted white chocolate. Put on a parchment paper–lined baking sheet and chill to set the chocolate.

HOMEMADE CHOCOLATE BARS

PALEO • GRAIN-FREE • VEGAN • NUT-FREE • NO-BAKE
GLUTEN-FREE • DAIRY-FREE

Since I discovered cacao butter as an ingredient, I've been making homemade chocolate bars galore. I had been making homemade chocolate with coconut oil but switched to cacao butter, which has a higher melting point. I discovered that I could actually bake with my homemade chocolate bars without them melting entirely into the baked good. The base of homemade chocolate is simple—it's just a combination of melted cacao butter, cacao powder, maple syrup or honey, and a pinch of salt. From there, the flavor combinations are endless! I provide four ideas on the next page, but use your imagination. Just about anything could be mixed in to create your own homemade chocolate bars. This would be tons of fun to make with kids!

Prep time: 10 minutes

Chill time: 1 hour

Total time: 1 hour 10 minutes

Yield: 2 or 3 chocolate bars, depending on size (about 2 cups chopped chocolate chunks)

½ cup (76g) coarsely chopped cacao butter

½ cup (42g) cacao powder or cocoa powder

2 to 3 tablespoons (42g to 63g) pure maple syrup or honey

Pinch of salt

IN a microwave-safe bowl, microwave the cacao butter in 30-second intervals, stirring between each, until completely melted, about 1 minute. Whisk in the cacao powder, 2 tablespoons of the maple syrup, and the salt until completely smooth. Taste and add more maple syrup if it's not sweet enough.

POUR the mixture into a chocolate bar mold (mine has two molds, each about 6 × 3 × ⅜ inches). If you don't have a chocolate mold, spread the chocolate in a small parchment paper–lined rimmed baking sheet, or divide among six muffin cups with paper liners. Refrigerate the chocolate bars until firm, about 1 hour. Remove the candy bars from their molds or pans and serve.

IF you made the bars in a mold, wrap the bars in plastic wrap or parchment paper for storage and serving. If the chocolate was spread on a small baking sheet, break it into shards. The chocolate will be in mounds if put in muffin cups. Store in a cool dry place or in the refrigerator for up to 1 month.

CONTINUES

Variations

These mix-ins are delicious, but they're also just suggestions! Feel free to be creative with yours to create your own custom chocolate bars. Play with different extracts, nuts, seeds, and dried fruits.

ALMOND–SEA SALT CHOCOLATE: Sprinkle a pinch of flaky sea salt on the bottom of each chocolate mold and add 10 to 12 roasted almonds before pouring the chocolate over it all.

PEPPERMINT-CACAO CHOCOLATE: Stir 2 tablespoons cacao nibs and ½ teaspoon peppermint extract into the melted chocolate.

FRUIT AND NUT CHOCOLATE: Add 2 tablespoons each dried fruit (chopped if large) and chopped nuts of your choice to the melted chocolate.

NUT BUTTER SWIRL CHOCOLATE: After pouring the chocolate into the mold or pan, swirl 1 heaping teaspoon melted nut butter into each chocolate bar mold. Choose your favorite nut butter.

CHOCOLATE-CARAMEL COOKIE BARS

PALEO • GRAIN-FREE • VEGAN • GLUTEN-FREE • DAIRY-FREE

The first time I bit into one of these bars—over four years ago when I had just gone all the way into gluten-free, dairy-free, and refined sugar-free baking—I was amazed at how they turned out. I was perplexed as to how just six simple ingredients could re-create one of my favorite candy bars, Twix. Over the years since, this recipe has been shared hundreds of thousands of times on social media, and I've heard from countless members of my blog community who continue to make the bars over and over again. The "caramel" is made from a magical mixture of nut butter, maple syrup, coconut oil, vanilla, and salt, and it will amaze you! I hope you love this recipe as much as I do!

PREHEAT the oven to 350°F. Lightly grease a 14 × 5-inch tart pan or an 8 × 8-inch baking pan with coconut oil. If the pan doesn't have a removable bottom, I also recommend lining it with parchment paper.

FOR THE SHORTBREAD: In a mixing bowl, stir together the coconut oil and maple syrup. Add the coconut flour and salt and stir, pressing out any clumps of coconut oil as you do.

PRESS the dough into the prepared pan as evenly as possible. Bake for 9 to 11 minutes, until light golden brown. Remove the pan from the oven and set on a wire rack until the shortbread is completely cool.

FOR THE FILLING: Combine all the filling ingredients in a small saucepan. Heat over medium-low heat until melted and completely mixed. Pour the filling over the crust and refrigerate until cool and set, 30 to 60 minutes.

FOR THE TOPPING: Whisk together the coconut oil, cocoa powder, and maple syrup until smooth, then pour over the set caramel layer. Smooth evenly and sprinkle with sea salt. Let the topping cool until set, about 20 minutes. Cut into 1-inch slices, or 16 squares. Refrigerate in an airtight container for up to 1 week.

Prep time: 20 minutes
Bake time: 9 minutes
Chill time: 50 minutes
Total time: 1 hour 20 minutes
Yield: about 16 squares or more, depending how they are cut

FOR THE SHORTBREAD CRUST

⅓ cup (67g) refined coconut oil, solid but softened

3 tablespoons (63g) pure maple syrup

⅔ cup (86g) coconut flour

Pinch of kosher salt

FOR THE CARAMEL FILLING

½ cup (128g) creamy cashew butter (almond butter or any other nut/seed butter of your choice can also be used)

⅓ cup (113g) pure maple syrup

⅓ cup (67g) refined coconut oil, melted

1 teaspoon pure vanilla extract

¼ teaspoon kosher salt

FOR THE CHOCOLATE TOPPING

¼ cup (50g) refined coconut oil, melted

¼ cup (21g) cocoa powder

2 tablespoons (42g) pure maple syrup

¼ teaspoon flaky sea salt (optional)

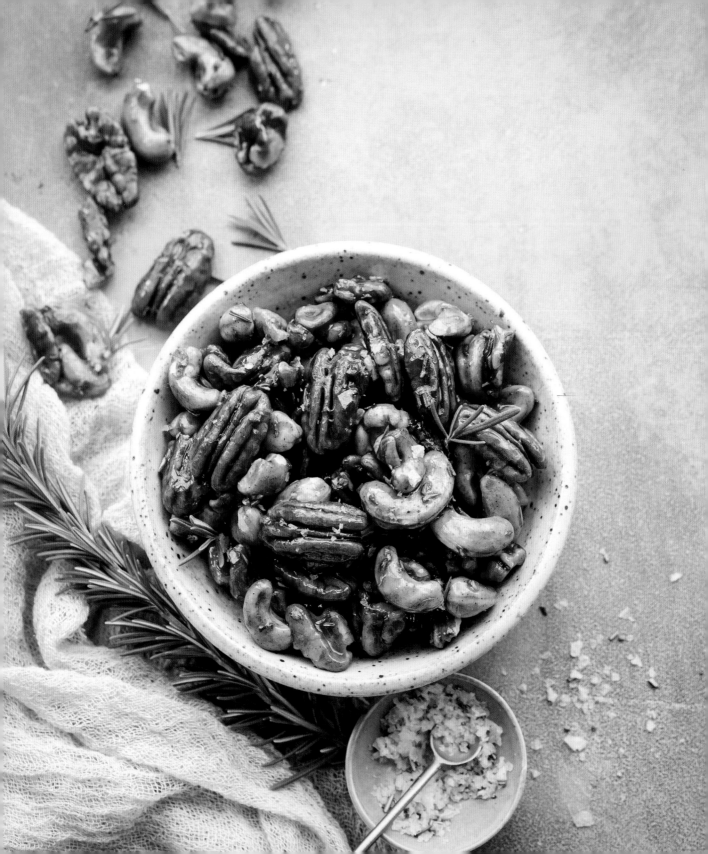

ROSEMARY-SPICED CANDIED NUTS

PALEO • GRAIN-FREE • VEGAN • NO-BAKE • GLUTEN-FREE • DAIRY-FREE

Candied nuts are best around the holidays. They're perfect for filling bowls to set out with the desserts, and make a beautiful sweet addition to any snack board. They're also great chopped up and used to adorn other treats. I always assumed you'd need white sugar to get that snappy shell that surrounds the best candied nuts, but it turns out that honey and maple syrup do the trick! I use a combo of the two liquid sweeteners so neither flavor overpowers the other, but you can use all of one or the other if you prefer. The additions of cinnamon, cayenne, and fresh rosemary make these more interesting and delicious than plain candied nuts, helping to cut through the sweetness and adding a spicy, herbaceous depth of flavor.

Prep time: 5 minutes
Cook time: 20 minutes
Total time: 25 minutes
Yield: about 3 cups

¼ cup (85g) pure maple syrup

2 tablespoons (42g) pure honey (or use 2 additional tablespoons maple syrup instead to keep these nuts vegan)

1 teaspoon ground cinnamon

¼ teaspoon kosher salt

⅛ to ¼ teaspoon cayenne pepper

2 cups (226g) raw mixed nuts

2 teaspoons chopped fresh rosemary

LINE a baking sheet with parchment paper and grease lightly with coconut oil.

IN a heavy-bottomed saucepan, combine the maple syrup, honey, cinnamon, salt, and ⅛ teaspoon cayenne. Whisk to combine and bring to a boil over medium-high heat, stirring frequently. When the mixture starts boiling, add the nuts and turn the heat down to medium-low. Add more cayenne if you like a little more heat. Let the syrup cook for about 20 minutes, stirring frequently, until reduced and the nuts are coated completely. You shouldn't see any syrup pooling around or below the nuts, but each nut will have a thin candied layer. Stir in the chopped rosemary.

TO test if the nuts are ready, put one or two nuts in the freezer for 1 to 2 minutes. If the coating on the nuts is firm and forms a snappy shell, they're done. If the nuts are still a little sticky, cook them for a few more minutes.

POUR the candied nuts onto the prepared baking sheet and spread them out in an even layer. Let them cool completely at room temperature. Store in an airtight container at room temperature for up to 4 days.

Prep time: 20 minutes

Chill time: 30 minutes

Total time: 50 minutes

Yield: 12 peanut butter cups

FOR THE CHOCOLATE

½ cup (76g) coarsely chopped cacao butter

½ cup (42g) cacao powder

¼ cup (85g) pure maple syrup

Pinch of kosher salt

FOR THE PEANUT BUTTER FILLING

1 cup (256g) creamy natural peanut butter

1 tablespoon coconut flour

2 tablespoons (42g) pure maple syrup

¼ teaspoon kosher salt (skip if the peanut butter is salted)

CHOCOLATE–PEANUT BUTTER CUPS

GRAIN-FREE • VEGAN • NO-BAKE • GLUTEN-FREE • DAIRY-FREE

Chocolate–peanut butter cups have had my heart for a long time. My dad and I obsess about all things chocolate and peanut butter, as he turned me on to loving the combination. Peanut butter cups were always the most accessible way to devour the duo. This recipe sets out to replicate the orange-wrapped candy that was ever-present during my childhood, but with more wholesome ingredients. We've got a quick and easy homemade chocolate coating and a simple, lightly sweetened peanut butter filling. I like storing a stash of these in my refrigerator for whenever I'm craving a little sweet peanut butter treat!

LINE a muffin tin with twelve paper liners.

FOR THE CHOCOLATE: Chop the cacao butter into even finer pieces and put in a microwave-safe bowl. Microwave in 20-second intervals, stirring between each, until fully melted. The cacao butter can also be melted over a double boiler set over medium-low heat.

ADD the cacao powder, maple syrup, and salt and stir until smooth. Pour a small amount of the mixture into the bottom of each paper liner to cover the bottom. Don't use more than half the chocolate for this. Tilt the pan slightly in all directions to partially coat the sides of each liner with chocolate, but most of the chocolate should be on the bottom of the liner. Set aside the remaining melted chocolate.

FOR THE FILLING: In a mixing bowl, stir together the peanut butter, coconut flour, maple syrup, and salt until the mixture is smooth and holds together as a dough. Scoop out a slightly rounded tablespoon of the dough and roll into a ball. Flatten the ball between your palms into a disc about 1¾ inches in diameter. Put the disc in the center of the chocolate in one of the paper liners, pressing it down into the chocolate so the chocolate covers the sides. Repeat until all of the liners are filled with a peanut butter disc and the sides of each disc are coated with chocolate.

POUR enough of the reserved chocolate mixture over the peanut butter discs to cover them completely. If at any point the reserved melted chocolate thickens, warm it in the microwave for 10 to 15 seconds until it's fluid.

REFRIGERATE the peanut butter cups for at least 30 minutes to firm up. Store at cool room temperature or in an airtight container in the refrigerator.

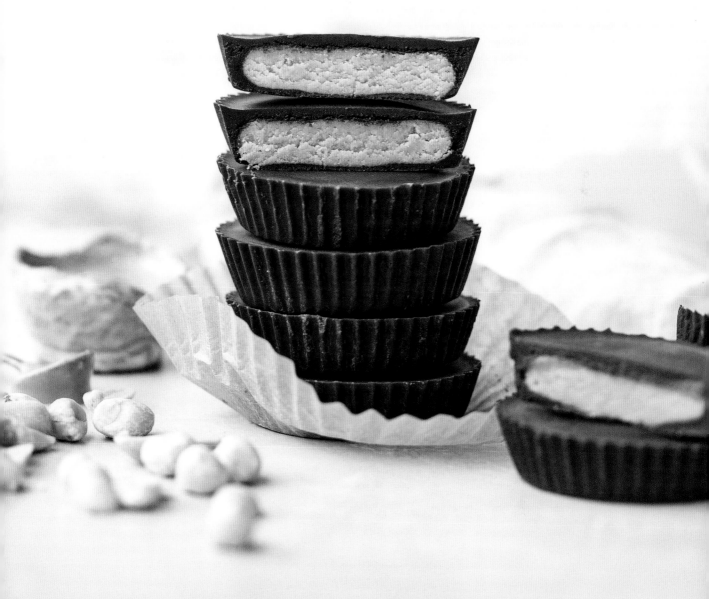

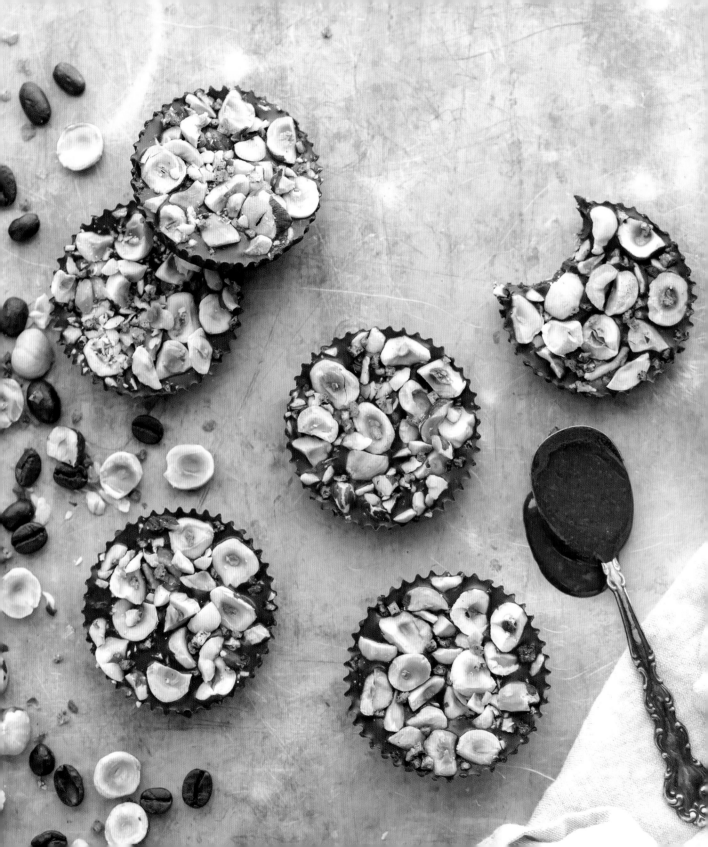

MOCHA HAZELNUT FUDGE

PALEO • GRAIN-FREE • VEGAN • NO-BAKE • GLUTEN-FREE • DAIRY-FREE

What's even better than chocolate and hazelnut together? Adding espresso powder for a mocha hazelnut treat that will make any hazelnut lover's mouth water. The sweet, creamy fudge base gets loaded up with homemade chocolate hazelnut butter to help keep it creamy, along with a hearty dose of espresso powder for a coffee-flavored boost. Hazelnuts and sea salt on top add crunch. If you avoid caffeine, simply leave out the espresso powder or seek out decaf espresso powder.

COMBINE the cacao butter and coconut oil in a 2-cup liquid measuring cup or similar microwave-safe container. Microwave in 20-second intervals, stirring between each, until the mixture is fully melted, about 1 minute. It can also be melted in a double boiler, if you prefer. Transfer to a bowl for easy mixing.

ADD the cacao powder, hazelnut butter, maple syrup, espresso powder, and kosher salt. Whisk or stir until completely smooth, making sure to break up any clumps of cacao powder.

SCRAPE the fudge mixture into a small, parchment paper–lined pan, such as a loaf pan; or divide it evenly among twelve muffin pan cups, either silicone or metal, lined with paper liners. Garnish with the toasted hazelnuts and sea salt if using. Refrigerate for at least 1 hour to firm up. If made in a pan, cut the fudge into 12 to 24 pieces. Store in an airtight container in the refrigerator for up to 1 week.

Prep time: 10 minutes
Chill time: 1 hour
Total time: 1 hour 10 minutes
Yield: 12 to 24 pieces, depending on how they are cut

⅓ cup (51g) chopped cacao butter

1 tablespoon refined coconut oil, softened

¾ cup (72g) cacao powder

⅓ cup (85g) Chocolate Hazelnut Butter (page 269)

¼ cup (85g) pure maple syrup

1 tablespoon espresso powder

¼ teaspoon kosher salt

½ cup (57g) toasted hazelnuts, chopped

1 teaspoon flaky sea salt (optional but recommended)

Prep time: 15 minutes
Chill time: 2 hours
Total time: 2¼ hours
Yield: 18 pieces

FOR THE COOKIE DOUGH

1 cup (256g) cashew butter or other creamy nut butter of choice

¼ cup (85g) pure maple syrup

1 cup (96g) blanched almond flour

¼ cup (32g) coconut flour

¼ cup (25g) mini chocolate chips (see Tip), plus more for sprinkling

1 teaspoon pure vanilla extract

¼ teaspoon kosher salt

FOR THE CHOCOLATE TOPPING

4 ounces bittersweet chocolate, chopped or in chips (about ⅔ cup)

2 tablespoons (32g) cashew butter, or the nut butter used in the cookie dough

½ teaspoon flaky sea salt (optional)

Tip

I like Enjoy Life mini chocolate chips. If you want less sugar and are following a Paleo diet, substitute cacao nibs for the chocolate chips.

COOKIE DOUGH FUDGE

NO-BAKE • PALEO • GRAIN-FREE • VEGAN • GLUTEN-FREE • DAIRY-FREE

Anything cookie dough–related brings to mind my best friend since elementary school, Paige. We used to spend hours baking together when we were growing up and she always shamelessly stole spoonfuls of cookie dough before we could get it onto the baking sheet. This Cookie Dough Fudge re-creates the cookie dough we used to sneak from the mixing bowl, but gives it an egg-free makeover. Instead of spoons, this is cookie dough you can pick up and walk around with as it won't melt in your hands. But it will give you that same sweet doughy satisfaction—complete with the crunch of chocolate chips. If you're a fellow cookie dough stealer, these are a must try.

LINE a 9 × 5-inch loaf pan with parchment paper and grease the paper lightly with coconut oil.

FOR THE COOKIE DOUGH: In a small mixing bowl, stir together the nut butter and maple syrup. Stir in the almond flour, coconut flour, chocolate chips, vanilla, and kosher salt. Press into the prepared pan in as even a layer as possible.

FOR THE CHOCOLATE TOPPING: In a microwave-safe bowl, microwave the chocolate and nut butter for 30 seconds and then stir. Microwave for another 30 seconds and stir again. The chocolate should be soft and shiny and melt when stirred. Repeat if necessary, until the chocolate and butter are smooth and completely blended. Spread the chocolate topping evenly over the cookie dough layer as evenly as possible.

SPRINKLE with sea salt if using and more mini chocolate chips, if desired, and refrigerate until firm, at least 2 hours. Once firm, cut into 18 squares. Refrigerate in an airtight container for 2 weeks; or wrap well in plastic and freeze in a freezer-safe plastic bag for up to 3 months.

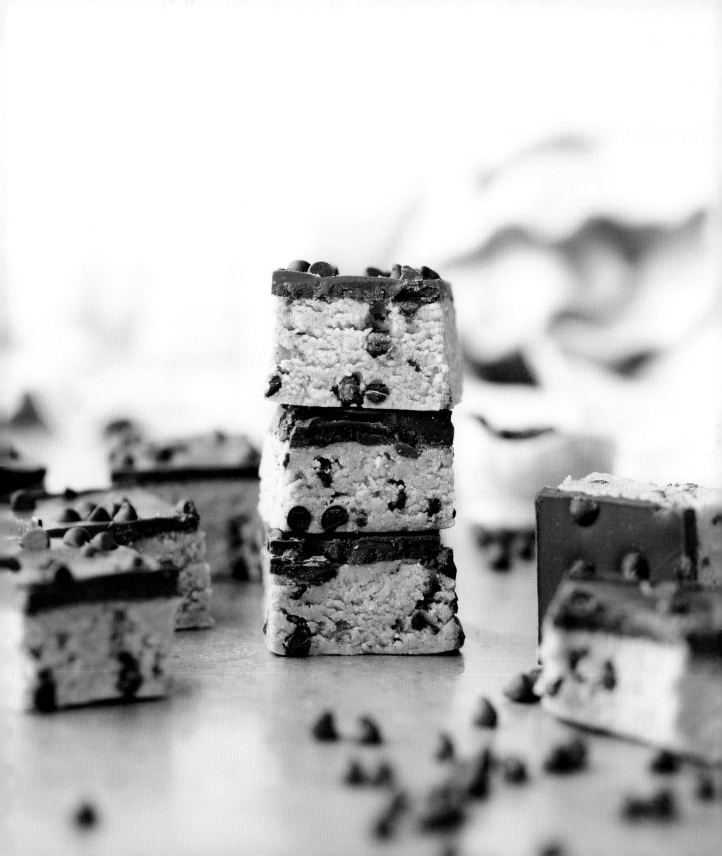

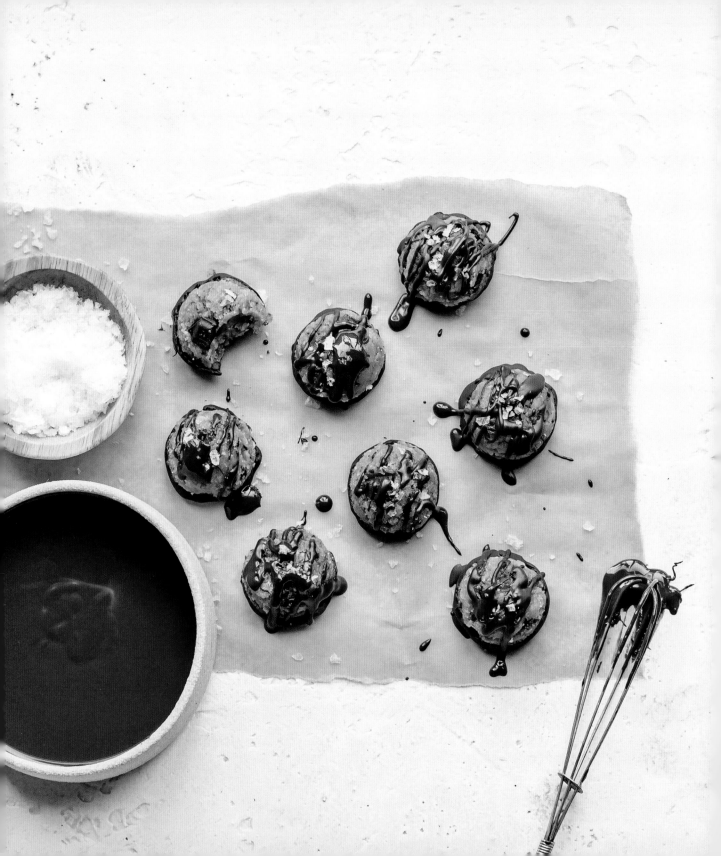

CHOCOLATE CHIP COOKIE DOUGH BITES

PALEO • GRAIN-FREE • VEGAN • NO-BAKE • GLUTEN-FREE • DAIRY-FREE

Ever made a batch of cookie dough just for the purpose of eating the dough straight out of the bowl? Yeah, me too. If you're the type, you're going to love these cookie dough bites. All the flavor and texture you love about cookie dough, intentionally made to be devoured by the spoonful . . . or if you've got the patience, to be scooped, and then dunked and drizzled with more chocolate. I added some toasted pecans for a little extra crunch, but if you're in the anti-nuts-in-cookies camp, leave them out and add more chocolate chips.

FOR THE COOKIE DOUGH: Spread the pecans in a single layer in a dry skillet. Toast over medium heat, stirring frequently, until the nuts are aromatic and lightly browned, 3 to 4 minutes. Slide the toasted nuts from the pan onto a plate and let them cool.

IN a mixing bowl, stir together the coconut oil and coconut sugar until smooth. Add the flax egg, vanilla, and sea salt and stir until fully mixed. Add the almond flour and mix until well incorporated. Fold in the chocolate chips and toasted pecans.

FROM here, you can enjoy the dough with a spoon, or make cute chocolate-dunked truffles.

FOR truffles, cover a plate or small baking sheet with parchment paper. Use a small cookie scoop (mine holds 2 teaspoons of dough) or a spoon to form balls of dough to resemble truffles. Put them on the prepared plate and refrigerate for about 20 minutes to firm up, or freeze for about 10 minutes.

FOR THE CHOCOLATE DIP: Once the truffles are firm, put the chocolate in a small, microwave-safe bowl and microwave for 45 seconds. Stir and melt for another 30 seconds. Microwave for 20 seconds longer, if necessary, stirring the chocolate until it's smooth and fluid.

Prep time: 10 minutes
Chill time: 30 minutes
Total time: 40 minutes
Yield: 20 cookie dough bites

FOR THE COOKIE DOUGH
¼ cup (28g) chopped pecans
¼ cup (50g) refined coconut oil, softened
¼ cup (36g) coconut sugar
½ flax egg (see Tip)
1 teaspoon pure vanilla extract
¼ teaspoon sea salt
1¼ cups (120g) blanched almond flour
2 ounces bittersweet chocolate chips or bittersweet chocolate, chopped (about ⅓ cup)

FOR THE CHOCOLATE DIP
3 ounces bittersweet chocolate chips or bittersweet chocolate, chopped (about 6 tablespoons)
Flaky sea salt, for sprinkling (optional)

Tip

To make ½ flax egg, whisk 1½ teaspoons ground flax seed with 1½ tablespoons water. Let set for 10 minutes to give it time to gel.

CONTINUES

USING a fork or dipping tool, dip the bottom of each truffle into the chocolate and let the excess drip off before returning the truffles to the parchment-covered plate. Repeat until all are dipped and have a chocolate base.

TRANSFER the remaining chocolate to a piping bag or zippered plastic bag with a corner snipped off. Drizzle the remaining chocolate over the truffles. You can also drizzle with a spoon. Sprinkle with flaky sea salt, if desired.

BEFORE serving, return the truffles to the refrigerator or freezer to firm up the chocolate, about 10 minutes. Store in an airtight container for up to 1 week in the refrigerator, or up to 3 months in the freezer.

PALEO VANILLA-BEAN MARSHMALLOWS

PALEO • GRAIN-FREE • NO-BAKE • GLUTEN-FREE • DAIRY-FREE

I still remember the first time I made marshmallows back when I was seventeen. It was the first time I'd ever worked with gelatin and one of my first times ever boiling sugar syrup, and I was terrified about all of it. But magically, as I beat the sugar syrup into the bloomed gelatin, it transformed from a sticky liquid into puffy white clouds of marshmallow fluff. I ended up with marshmallow fluff in my hair, on my shirt, and somehow, on my sneakers, but the results were transformative. There's no going back once you've tried a homemade marshmallow: It's fluffier and more delicious than any you can buy in the store. These Paleo marshmallows are made with a combination of honey and maple syrup, speckled with vanilla bean powder, and are somehow not nearly as sticky as their white sugar–filled counterparts. Best part? They toast beautifully for s'mores, especially when paired with Homemade Graham Crackers (page 173) and Homemade Chocolate Bars (page 231)! I also include an option to make them a dessert in their own right, with a dunk in dark chocolate and a sprinkling of flaky sea salt.

CHOOSE an 8×8-inch square baking pan (for thick marshmallows), a 9×9-inch pan (for slightly thinner), or a 9×13-inch pan (for thin marshmallows) and grease very well with coconut oil, using a paper towel to rub it in and making sure you fully coat the bottom, sides, and corners of the pan. Set aside.

IN the bowl of a stand mixer fitted with the whisk attachment, combine the gelatin and ½ cup of the cold water, whisking gently to combine. Let it stand while you make the sugar syrup to allow the gelatin to bloom and thicken.

IN a deep, medium saucepan, combine the honey, maple syrup, and remaining ½ cup water. Stir gently and then clip a candy thermometer on the pan so that it is submerged in the syrup but not touching the bottom of the pan. Bring the syrup to a boil and cook, stirring or whisking occasionally, until it reaches 235°F to

CONTINUES

Prep time: 30 minutes

Cook time: 30 minutes

Total time: 1 hour (plus 6 hours for setting)

Yield: about 36 marshmallows, depending how they are cut

- 3 tablespoons unflavored gelatin (see Tip)
- 1 cup cold water
- ¾ cup (255g) honey
- ½ cup (170g) pure maple syrup
- 1 tablespoon pure vanilla extract
- ¾ teaspoon vanilla bean powder, or ½ vanilla bean, scraped
- ¼ teaspoon kosher salt
- About ¼ cup tapioca flour, for dusting
- 3 ounces bittersweet chocolate, chopped (about 6 tablespoons), for dipping (optional)
- Flaky sea salt, for sprinkling (optional)

Tip

When it comes to gelatin, I like to make sure to use grass-fed gelatins.

240°F (soft-ball stage). This takes 30 to 40 minutes. Once the syrup reaches 240°F, remove the pan from the heat.

TURN the mixer to medium speed and slowly pour the hot sugar syrup into the gelatin mixture. When all the syrup has been added, turn the speed to medium-high and whisk until the marshmallow is white and fluffy, 8 to 10 minutes. Add the vanilla extract, vanilla bean powder, and kosher salt and mix for 30 seconds longer.

POUR the marshmallow into the prepared pan. Use an offset spatula that's been greased with coconut oil to even it out. Tap the pan on the counter a few times to get rid of air bubbles. Let the marshmallow sit at room temperature for about 6 hours or until firm. (I usually leave it overnight.)

USE a knife to loosen the marshmallow from the edges of the pan and invert it onto a tapioca flour-dusted work surface. Dust the marshmallow slab with more tapioca flour and cut it into whatever size pieces you wish (a pizza cutter works great here). Dip the sticky edges of the marshmallows in more tapioca flour and then shake in a fine-mesh sieve to remove excess.

OPTIONALLY, you can dip half of the marshmallows in melted dark chocolate (or the whole marshmallows!) and sprinkle them with sea salt. Microwave the dark chocolate in a microwave-safe bowl in 30-second intervals, stirring between each, until fully melted. Dip half of each marshmallow into the chocolate and place on a parchment-lined baking sheet. Sprinkle with flaky sea salt and transfer to the fridge to harden. Store the marshmallows in an airtight container at room temperature for up to 1 week.

Variation

After pouring the marshmallow mixture into the pan to set, you can sprinkle the top with chopped nuts, cacao nibs, dried fruit, and anything else you can think of. There are lots of options! You also could use peppermint or orange extract instead of or along with the vanilla extract.

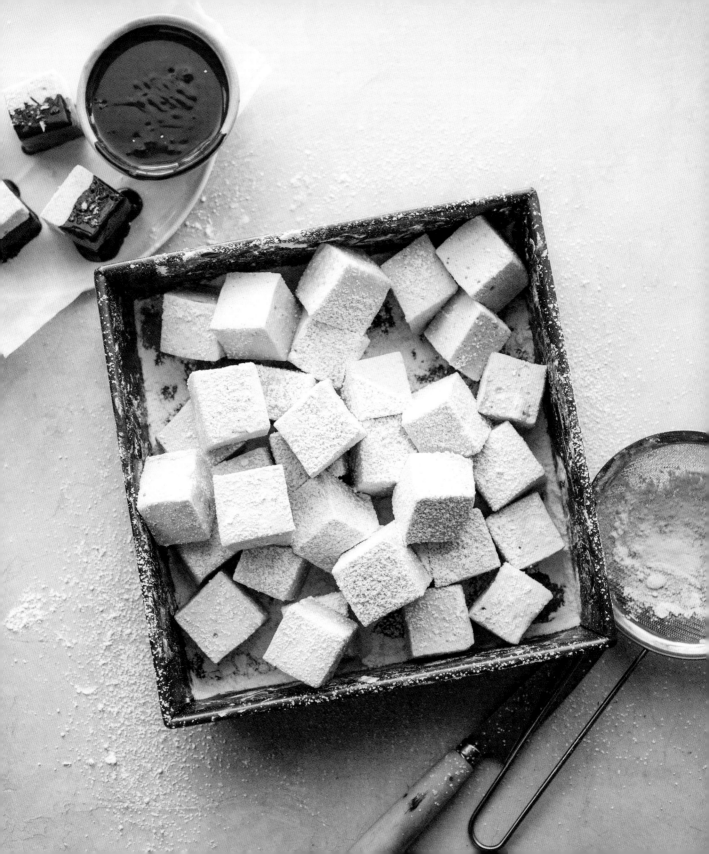

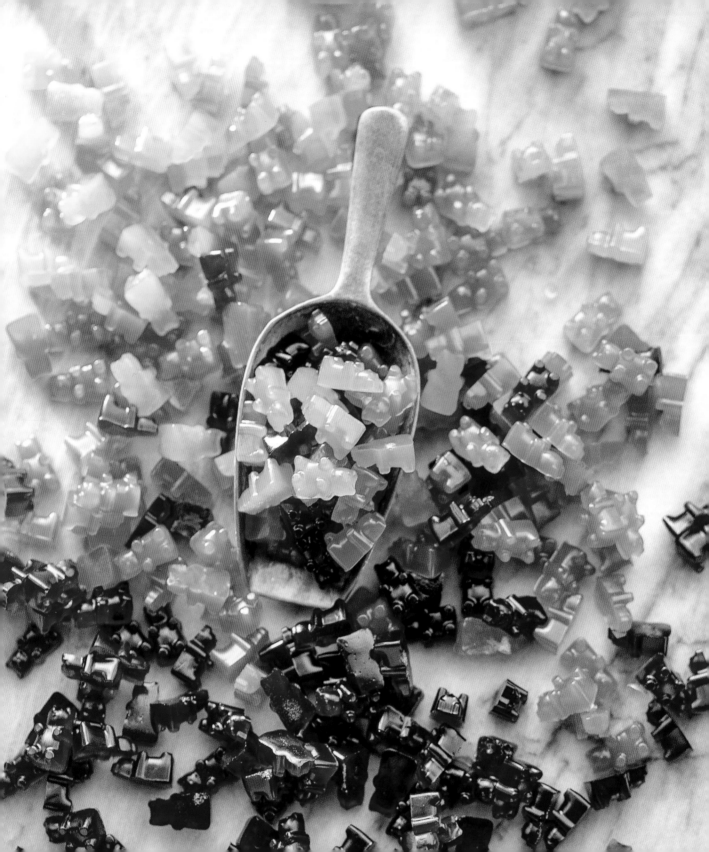

HOMEMADE GUMMY BEARS

PALEO • GRAIN-FREE • NO-BAKE • GLUTEN-FREE • DAIRY-FREE

When you want to see pure delight in someone's eyes, serve them a pile of homemade gummy bears. With wide eyes, people will gasp, "You made these?" You get to say yes, knowing how easy it was, with only a few simple ingredients. These gummies are not exactly like the ones you get in the store. They're not quite as chewy, but they have a melt-in-your-mouth quality that is juicy and delicious. For firmness, I use gelatin—make sure yours is grass-fed and sourced from a reputable company. I provide instructions for vegan gummies using agar powder in the Tips, but they tend to have a softer texture than ones made with gelatin. For the molds, I found a set of two, each holding fifty gummies, on Amazon. The set comes with a dropper, making it super easy to fill the bear-shaped cavities. These are tons of fun to make with kids!

Prep time: 30 minutes

Chill time: 10 minutes

Total time: 40 minutes

Yield: 200 gummy bears

1 cup pure apple juice

2 to 3 tablespoons pure maple syrup or honey

Up to 1 tablespoon cinnamon extract (optional; see Tips)

4 tablespoons grass-fed gelatin

FOR APPLE-CINNAMON GUMMIES (SEE VARIATIONS FOR OTHER OPTIONS): In a small saucepan, combine the apple juice and 2 tablespoons of the maple syrup and heat over medium heat until steaming hot but not yet boiling.

REDUCE the heat to the lowest setting and stir in the cinnamon extract if using. Carefully taste the mixture and add more syrup or honey if needed. Whisk in the gelatin, 1 tablespoon at a time, making sure each tablespoon is fully dissolved in the liquid before adding the next.

ONCE the gelatin is fully dissolved, remove the pan from the heat and use a dropper to fill gummy bear molds. Refrigerate to firm up completely, 10 to 15 minutes if the molds are small. Once the gummies are firm, pop the gummy bears from the molds.

IF you have liquid left over after filling the molds, pour it into a small pan and let it harden in the refrigerator to firm up, then cut into squares. Alternatively, wait until the first gummies set, then gently reheat the mixture over low heat to liquefy, and refill the molds.

STORE the gummies in a sealed container in the refrigerator for up to 1 month.

CONTINUES

Variations

These flavor combinations are just fun suggestions! You can use any kind of juice you like, or even kombucha, to make these totally customizable.

POMEGRANATE GUMMIES: Instead of apple juice, use 1 cup pure pomegranate juice. Omit the cinnamon extract.

CRANBERRY-ORANGE GUMMIES: Instead of apple juice, use 1 cup pure orange juice plus 2 tablespoons pure cranberry juice. Omit the cinnamon extract.

CITRUS GUMMIES: Instead of apple juice, use ¾ cup pure orange juice plus 3 tablespoons fresh lemon juice. Omit the cinnamon extract.

Tips

- Different brands of cinnamon extract can vary in strength. I'd recommend starting with about ¾ tablespoon, tasting the mixture, and then adding more to your taste. If you're using pure cinnamon oil, it will be a lot stronger. Start with just 1 teaspoon and add more to taste.
- To make these vegan, replace the gelatin with 1 tablespoon plus 1 teaspoon agar powder for each cup of juice. Instead of adding the agar powder at the end of boiling as you do with the gelatin, mix it with the juice before you bring it to a simmer. Whisk frequently while the mixture simmers until it is thickened and syrupy, about 5 minutes, then add the sweetener and use the dropper to fill the molds.

CHOCOLATE FUDGE

PALEO • GRAIN-FREE • VEGAN • NO-BAKE • GLUTEN-FREE • DAIRY-FREE

This five-ingredient fudge has been a longtime favorite around here, for a couple of good reasons: It takes a quick 5 minutes to put together and when you bite into the creamy fudge, your teeth sink right in and it melts in your mouth. Also, the topping options are pretty much endless—I share a few variations, but use your imagination! All sorts of nuts, dried fruits, natural extracts, and more can be used to customize this simple fudge to fit your tastes. Because its creamy, melty qualities come from coconut oil, it's best not to let the fudge get too warm or else the coconut oil will start to melt, so make sure to keep this fudge stored in the refrigerator!

Prep time: 5 minutes
Chill time: 2 hours
Total time: about 2 hours
Yield: 18 pieces

- ½ cup (100g) refined coconut oil
- ¾ cup (63g) cocoa powder (preferably Dutch-processed)
- ¾ cup (192g) creamy almond butter, or nut butter of choice
- ⅓ cup (113g) pure maple syrup or honey
- 1 teaspoon pure vanilla extract (optional)
- ⅛ teaspoon kosher salt (optional)
- Flaky sea salt, for garnish (optional)

LINE a 9 × 5-inch loaf pan or other small baking pan with foil or parchment paper. The size of the loaf pan will determine the thickness of the fudge. An 8 × 8-inch pan will yield thinner fudge. You can also use a muffin tin; line 12 cups with paper liners.

MELT the coconut oil in a saucepan over medium-low heat or in the microwave for 30 to 60 seconds. Stir in the cocoa powder, nut butter, maple syrup, and, if using, the vanilla and kosher salt until completely smooth.

POUR the fudge into the prepared pan. If desired, garnish with flaky sea salt and/or other toppings (see the topping options on the next page). Refrigerate until chilled and firm, about 2 hours.

USING a sharp knife, cut the fudge into squares. Store in the refrigerator for up to 1 month.

CONTINUES

Topping Options

BERRIES: Diced strawberries are one of my favorite fudge toppings, but any berry will work! Top the fudge with 1 cup diced strawberries, blueberries, or raspberries, then drizzle with melted chocolate, if desired.

PEANUT BUTTER (PICTURED): Use peanut butter when making the fudge; then melt 2 tablespoons peanut butter with 1 tablespoon coconut oil, whisk, and drizzle over the fudge mixture once it's in the pan. Swirl the peanut butter mixture into the fudge with a knife or toothpick. This can be done with any other nut or seed butter as well.

PEPPERMINT: Add 1 teaspoon pure peppermint extract with the vanilla extract. Top the fudge with 2 tablespoons crushed peppermint candies or candy canes (preferably naturally colored and flavored).

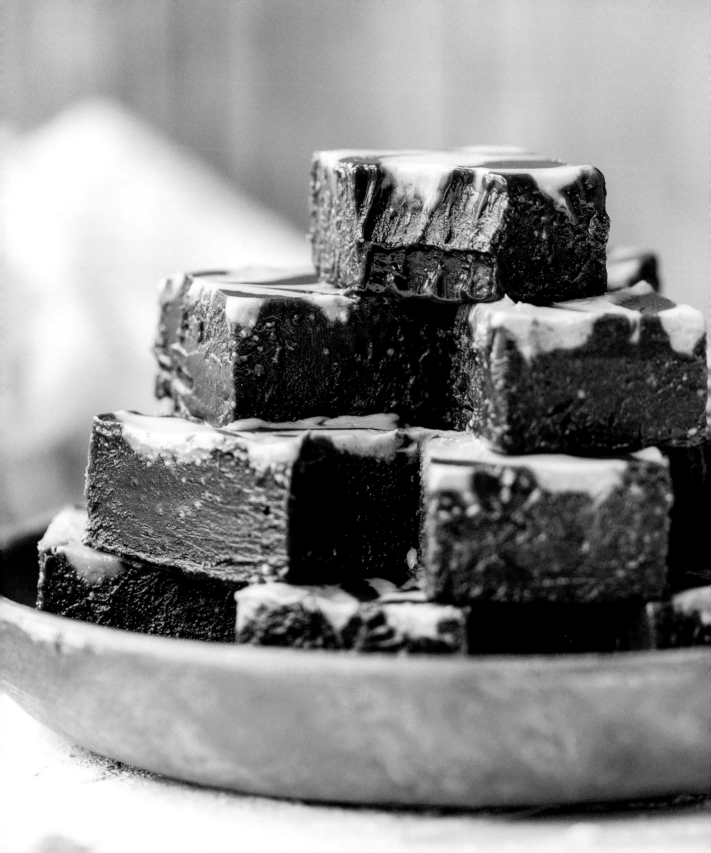

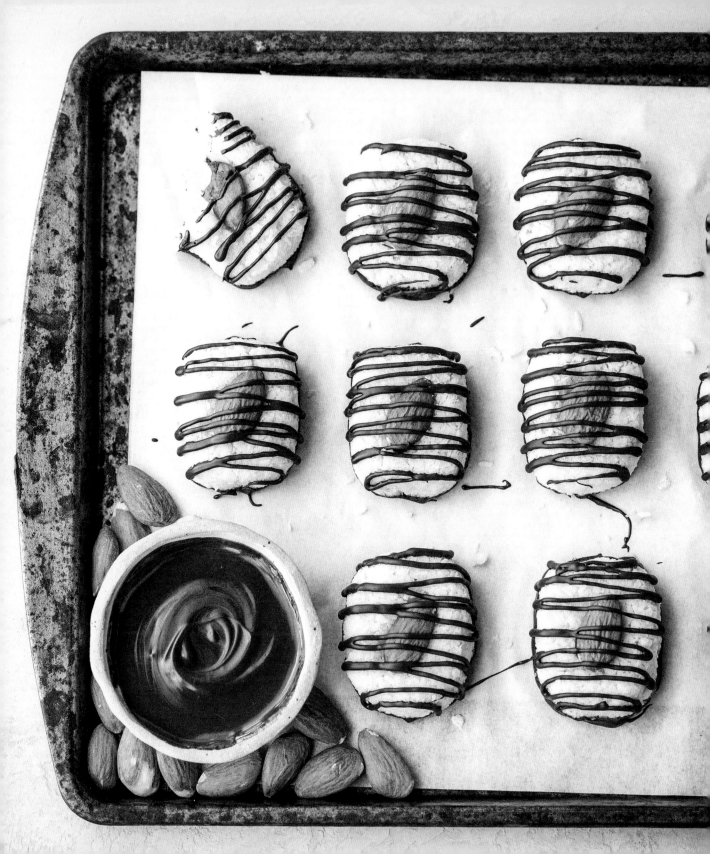

HOMEMADE ALMOND DELIGHTS

PALEO • GRAIN-FREE • VEGAN • NO-BAKE • GLUTEN-FREE • DAIRY-FREE

I went on a kick re-creating some of my favorite classic candy for this book, like the Chocolate-Caramel Cookie Bars (page 233), Crunchy Bars (page 227), and Chocolate–Peanut Butter Cups (page 236). I couldn't leave out one of my mom's all-time favorites: Almond Joy! So, almond delights were born. A scrumptious combination of coconut and almonds, lightly sweetened and dunked in chocolate, they will satisfy any coconut lovers. If you were a bigger fan of this candy's almond-free cousin, feel free to skip the nuts!

Prep time: 30 minutes

Chill time: 1 hour

Total time: 1½ hours

Yield: 13 to 14 bars

3 tablespoons (63g) pure maple syrup

½ cup canned coconut cream

2 tablespoons (25g) refined coconut oil, melted

1½ cups (90g) coconut, finely shredded

About 14 whole almonds

4 ounces bittersweet chocolate, chopped (about ⅔ cup)

IN a mixing bowl, whisk together the maple syrup, coconut cream, and 1 tablespoon of the melted coconut oil. Stir in the coconut and mix until it is fully coated.

USING a small cookie scoop or spoon, divide the dough into 13 or 14 scoops. Arrange the scoops of dough on a parchment paper–lined baking sheet.

USING your hands, form each ball into a small rectangle. Top each rectangle with an almond and press it gently into the dough. Refrigerate for at least 30 minutes to firm up.

COMBINE the chocolate and remaining 1 tablespoon coconut oil in a microwave-safe bowl and microwave for about 30 seconds, stirring every 30 seconds, until the mixture is smooth and fluid.

DIP the bottom of each coconut bar into the chocolate, scraping off the excess chocolate. Return the bars to the parchment-lined baking sheet.

SCRAPE the remaining chocolate into a plastic zippered bag with the corner snipped off or a piping bag. Drizzle the chocolate over the bars.

REFRIGERATE again for at least 30 minutes to firm up the chocolate before enjoying! Store the bars in an airtight container in the refrigerator for up to 1 week.

Prep time: 20 minutes
Chill time: 45 minutes
Total time: 20 minutes
Yield: 18 truffles

....

6 pitted Medjool dates

¾ cup (192g) creamy peanut
    butter or another creamy nut
    or seed butter

½ cup (64g) coconut flour

2 to 4 tablespoons hot water

1 teaspoon pure vanilla extract

6 ounces bittersweet chocolate,
    finely chopped (about 1 cup)

Flaky sea salt, for garnish
    (optional)

CHOCOLATE–PEANUT BUTTER TRUFFLES

GRAIN-FREE • VEGAN • NO-BAKE • GLUTEN-FREE • DAIRY-FREE

Medjool dates are magical little fruits that, when blended with nut butter and coconut flour, make a delightfully chewy, candy-like bite. That's just how these chocolate peanut butter truffles are made, with no sweetener needed except for the dates. The truffles are then dunked in a coating of chocolate, needing only five ingredients for the whole dessert—plus some flaky sea salt on top if you're into that (I am). If you want to switch things up, use your favorite nut or seed butter in place of the peanut butter for your own unique dessert. Using a seed butter, like tahini or sunflower seed butter, will keep these nut-free as well!

....

LINE a plate or baking sheet with parchment paper.

IF the dates are not soft and pliable, soak in about 1 cup hot water for about 10 minutes to soften. Drain the dates.

IN a high-powered blender (I use a Vitamix) or bowl of a food processor fitted with the metal blade, blend the dates, peanut butter, coconut flour, 2 tablespoons of the hot water, and the vanilla. If the mixture is still a little dry, add the remaining 2 tablespoons hot water.

WITH a tablespoon, scoop 1 tablespoon of the peanut butter mixture, roll it into a ball, and put it on the prepared baking sheet. Repeat to make 18 truffles. Transfer to the freezer for 30 minutes to firm.

MEANWHILE, put the chopped chocolate in a small but deep microwave-safe bowl or cup. Microwave in 30-second intervals, stirring between each, until the chocolate is fully melted and smooth.

USING a fork or dipping tool, dip each ball in the melted chocolate to cover completely, letting the excess drip off before returning to the lined baking sheet. While the coating is still fluid on the truffles, sprinkle with flaky sea salt, if desired. Repeat until all the truffles are dipped, then put in the refrigerator to set, about 15 minutes.

STORE in an airtight container in the refrigerator for up to 2 weeks.

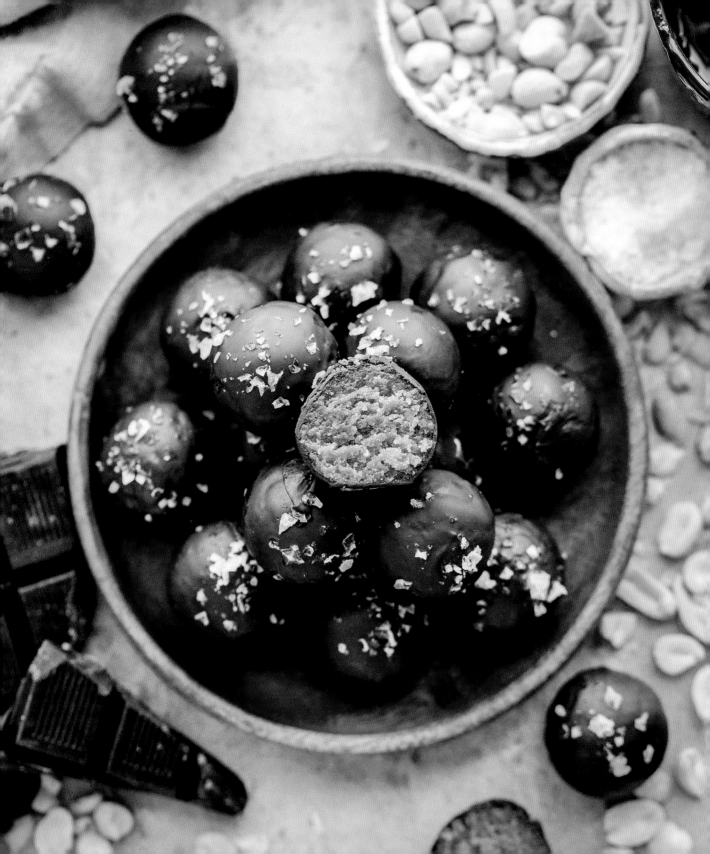

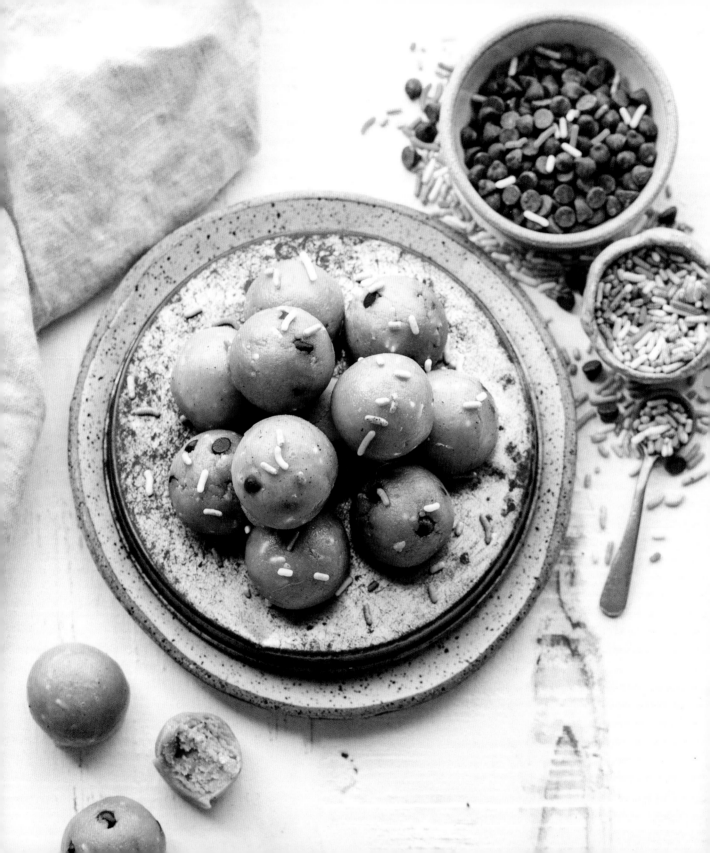

BIRTHDAY CAKE TRUFFLES

PALEO • GRAIN-FREE • VEGAN • NO-BAKE • GLUTEN-FREE • DAIRY-FREE

What if you could have all the flavor of birthday cake in cute little truffles, without the hassle of making a layer cake? I bet you'd make them—especially if it's as simple as this recipe! With raw cashew butter, maple syrup to sweeten, and almond and vanilla extracts for flavor, the easy truffle balls mimic the flavor of a vanilla birthday cake—sprinkles and all. The texture is similar to cookie dough. You can leave the truffles as they are, or dunk them in a sweet vanilla bean glaze, which firms up to form a delicious crust on the outside that crunches when you bite in, then melts on your tongue.

FOR THE TRUFFLES: In a mixing bowl, stir together the cashew butter and maple syrup. Stir in the almond flour, vanilla extract, almond extract, salt, and sprinkles.

USE a tablespoon to measure out each truffle and roll the dough into approximately 20 balls. Put them on a parchment paper–lined plate or tray. Refrigerate to firm up, about 10 minutes.

FOR THE GLAZE: Melt the cacao butter, coconut oil, and maple syrup in a small, deep bowl in the microwave for 30 seconds. Stir and microwave again in 15-second intervals, stirring between each, until fully melted. Whisk in the vanilla bean powder.

USING a fork or dipping tool, dip each truffle into the glaze, then let the excess drip off before returning to the plate. Stir the glaze as needed; the maple syrup and vanilla bean powder tend to sink to the bottom of the bowl without regular stirring.

FREEZE the truffles to allow them to firm up, about 10 minutes. Repeat until all the glaze is used, microwaving the glaze for 10 seconds if it begins to firm up. I glaze the balls three times each, letting the glaze firm up in the freezer between each dunk.

AFTER the last coating of glaze, while it still feels tacky, put the sprinkles in a shallow bowl and roll the truffles in them to coat, or just sprinkle them over the truffles.

STORE in an airtight container in the refrigerator for up to 1 month.

Prep time: 30 minutes
Chill time: 20 minutes
Total time: 50 minutes
Yield: 20 truffles

FOR THE TRUFFLES
- ½ cup (128g) raw cashew butter
- 3 tablespoons (63g) pure maple syrup
- 1 cup plus 2 tablespoons (108g) blanched almond flour
- 1 teaspoon pure vanilla extract
- ¾ teaspoon pure almond extract
- ¼ teaspoon kosher salt
- 3 tablespoons naturally-colored sprinkles

FOR THE GLAZE (OPTIONAL BUT RECOMMENDED)
- 2 tablespoons cacao butter, chopped finely if it's not already in chips
- 1 tablespoon refined coconut oil, softened
- 1 tablespoon pure maple syrup
- ⅛ teaspoon vanilla bean powder
- 3 to 4 tablespoons naturally colored sprinkles (optional)

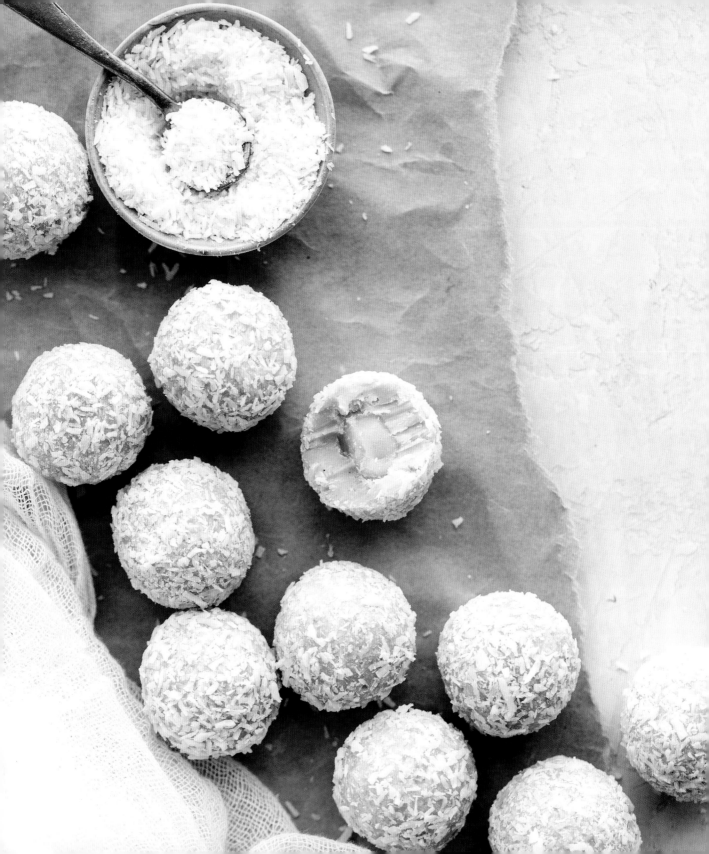

WHITE CHOCOLATE–COCONUT TRUFFLES

PALEO • GRAIN-FREE • VEGAN • NO-BAKE • GLUTEN-FREE • DAIRY-FREE

White chocolate isn't the easiest craving to satisfy when you're eating dairy-free: Milk is one of the main ingredients typically found in white chocolate and it helps provide the signature creaminess and white color. In this recipe, a combination of coconut milk and raw cashew butter provides the creaminess and structure, and cacao butter, maple syrup, and vanilla make it taste just like white chocolate. With a coconut coating and a macadamia nut tucked into the center of each, the truffles are elegant enough for gifting, but easy enough to keep a batch on hand all the time (and after you taste them, you'll want to!).

IN a microwave-safe bowl, mix the cacao butter with the coconut milk and maple syrup. Microwave for 1 minute, stirring every 30 seconds. If the truffle mixture is not fully melted after 1 minute, microwave in 15-second intervals until melted, stirring between each. You can also do this on the stove top over low heat.

WHISK in the cashew butter and vanilla. Refrigerate for 2 hours or until firm all the way through.

USE a small cookie scoop (I use a 2-teaspoon cookie scoop) or spoon to form small truffles, pressing a macadamia nut into the center of each before rolling it between your hands to form a ball that completely encases the nut.

SPREAD the coconut in a shallow bowl or rimmed plate. Roll each truffle in the coconut to coat. (Or you might want to drop the unformed truffles in the coconut before rolling them into balls. This way they don't soften between your palms.) Put on a plate or small baking sheet. Repeat until all the white chocolate mixture is rolled into truffles and coated. Refrigerate the truffles in an airtight container for up to 2 weeks.

Prep time: 30 minutes
Chill time: 2 hours
Total time: 2½ hours
Yield: 30 truffles

3 ounces cacao butter, chopped

¼ cup canned full-fat coconut milk

5 tablespoons (105g) pure maple syrup

½ cup (128g) raw cashew butter

1 teaspoon pure vanilla extract

30 toasted macadamia nuts (see Tip)

1 cup finely shredded coconut, plus more if necessary

Tip

You can use any nut you like in the middle of the truffle. My favorite is macadamia nuts, closely followed by hazelnuts.

CHAPTER SEVEN

Nut Butters, Sauces, and Beyond

A FEW TIPS AND TRICKS FOR SUCCESS:

If you're using a high-powered blender for grinding nut butters, it's important to use the tamper; I use the tamper almost continuously until the butter starts to smooth out and blend easily on its own. If using a food processor, you'll need to scrape down the sides frequently.

Some nuts are fattier than others, which will make the nut butter drippier. If you want the nut butter to be more drippy than solid, add coconut oil until it's the consistency you prefer.

Sometimes using vanilla extract in nut butters (or any liquid) can cause the nut butter to seize up. If that occurs, add coconut oil to thin it out.

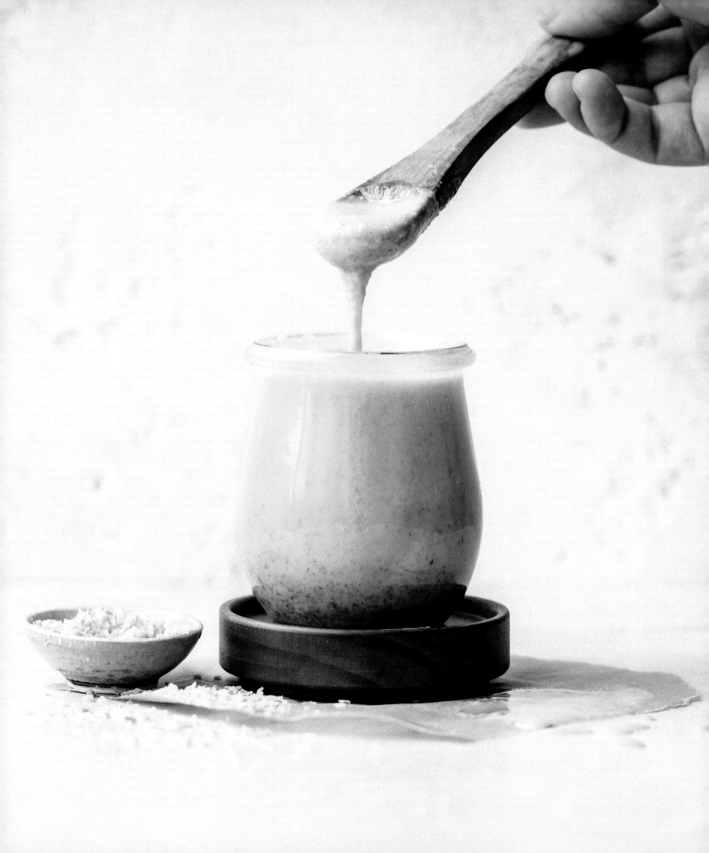

TOASTED COCONUT BUTTER

PALEO • GRAIN-FREE • VEGAN • NUT-FREE • NO-BAKE •
GLUTEN-FREE • DAIRY-FREE

A lot of recipes in this book use coconut butter as an ingredient,
but it's so delicious on its own and for dipping and drizzling. And it's
most delicious when the coconut flakes are first toasted until golden
brown and fragrant. This recipe is just one ingredient (coconut), with
possibly one more (coconut oil) if you need it. I wouldn't try making
a smaller batch—you need enough coconut in your blender or food
processor for it to break down properly. If you don't want it toasted,
skip that step and make raw coconut butter.

Prep time: 10 minutes
Bake time: 7 minutes
Total time: 17 minutes
Yield: about 1 cup

**4 cups (452g) unsweetened
shredded coconut (see Tip)**

**1 tablespoon virgin coconut oil,
melted (if needed)**

Tip

For a sweet and salty version,
add ⅛ teaspoon kosher salt
and 1 tablespoon coconut
sugar to the coconut butter
and blend it in.

PREHEAT the oven to 350°F.

SPREAD the coconut over a large baking sheet to create as even
a layer as possible. Bake for 7 to 10 minutes, stirring two or three
times, until the coconut turns golden brown. Slide the coconut off
the baking sheet onto a tray or plate to cool. Alternatively, spread
the coconut in a large skillet and cook over medium heat for 2 to
3 minutes, stirring almost constantly, until the coconut begins to
brown around the edges. Take the skillet from the heat and let the
coconut continue to brown in its ambient heat, stirring several times.

PUT the toasted coconut in a high-powered blender (I use a
Vitamix) or the bowl of a food processor fitted with the metal
blade.

WITH the machine on high, process the coconut to a smooth
butter. If you're using a high-powered blender, use the tamper
to push the coconut flakes down toward the blades until the
butter gets creamy enough to blend without it. It should take
3 to 5 minutes in the blender. If you're using a food processor,
scrape down the sides of the bowl frequently to ensure everything
is evenly blended. It will take between 6 to 12 minutes in the
processor. If the mixture seems dry after it's been blending for a
while, add the coconut oil to help it liquefy.

POUR the butter into a glass jar or container. It will be solid if
stored below 77°F. Microwave it for about 15 seconds or put the
sealed jar in a hot water bath to reliquefy.

Prep time: 10 minutes
Bake time: 10 minutes
Total time: 20 minutes
Yield: 2 cups

1½ cups (170g) raw almonds

1½ cups (170g) raw pecans

1 to 2 teaspoons ground
   cinnamon

⅛ to ¼ teaspoon sea salt

ADD-INS (CHOOSE 2 TO 5)
⅓ cup dried cranberries (try to
   get berries sweetened with
   apple juice)

¼ cup bittersweet chocolate
   chips

¼ cup shredded or flaked
   coconut, toasted if desired
   (see Tips)

¼ cup sliced almonds or
   chopped pecans

1 to 2 tablespoons chia seeds

1 to 2 tablespoons hemp seeds

1 to 2 tablespoons cacao nibs

TRAIL MIX NUT BUTTER
PALEO • GRAIN-FREE • VEGAN • NO-BAKE • GLUTEN-FREE • DAIRY-FREE

The inspiration for this recipe came from the Hillcrest Farmers Market, the local market I visit most Sundays to gather my produce and locally made goods for the week. There's a woodworker there who makes gorgeous wooden spoons and kitchenware, and whenever I (or anyone) stops to browse his beautiful wares, he pulls out a container filled with homemade apple chips and the most irresistible almond butter. The nut butter is full of nuts, seeds, and dried fruit, and the homemade apple chips dipped in the butter make the perfect snack. This is my take on his delicious nut butter. I made the recipe choose-your-own-adventure style, so you can customize the add-ins to your tastes and what you've got on hand.

PREHEAT the oven to 350°F.

SPREAD the almonds and pecans on a baking sheet. Roast the nuts for 10 to 12 minutes, until lightly browned and fragrant. Let the nuts cool completely.

WHEN cool, put the nuts in a high-powered blender or the bowl of a food processor fitted with the metal blade. (I like to use a Vitamix blender because it's faster.) Blend on medium-high speed, scraping down the sides of the blender and the bowl as necessary, until the nut mixture is smooth and liquefied. The blender will need about 2 minutes and the food processor will need closer to 10 minutes.

ONCE the nut butter is nice and fluid, slow down the machine to low and add the cinnamon and salt to taste. Pulse in the add-ins of choice just until incorporated. Do not overmix; you want the butter to be chunky.

STORE in a lidded glass jar or plastic container in the refrigerator for up to 1 month.

Tips

- You can vary the nuts to suit your tastes; almonds and pecans is my favorite combo! My favorite mix-in combo is cranberries, pecans, and 1 tablespoon each of hemp seeds, chia seeds, and cacao nibs.
- For toasted coconut, preheat the oven to 350°F and line a baking sheet with parchment paper. Add the coconut flakes or shreds and bake, stirring once in the middle of baking, for 3 to 5 minutes, until golden brown.

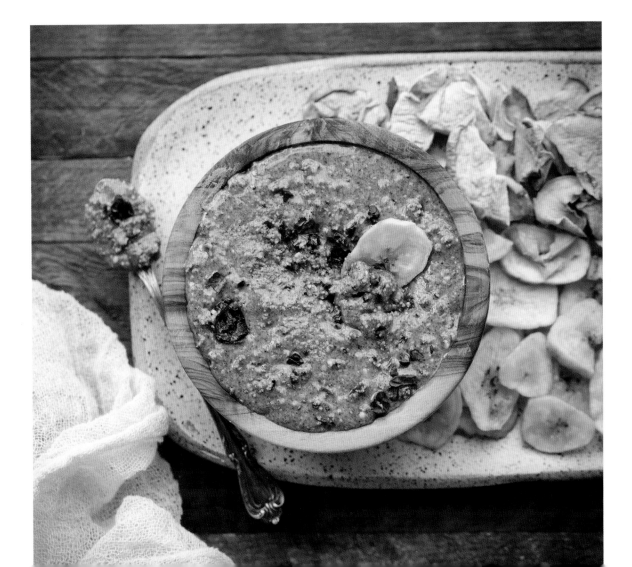

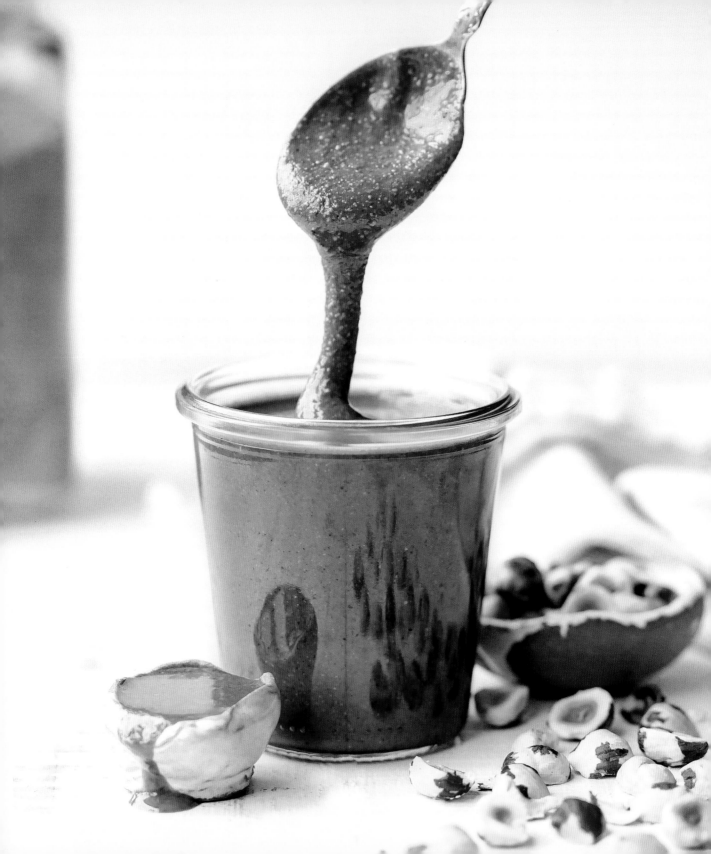

CHOCOLATE HAZELNUT BUTTER

PALEO • GRAIN-FREE • VEGAN • NO-BAKE • GLUTEN-FREE • DAIRY-FREE

I'm not going to say that this chocolate hazelnut butter tastes exactly like the ever-beloved Nutella, because it doesn't. But in my humble opinion, it's even better! You can actually taste the hazelnuts since the flavor isn't masked by loads of refined sugar, but it's still sweet and chocolatey enough to satisfy your sweet tooth. This recipe turned me into a true hazelnut lover! It's the perfect consistency for drizzling all over your oatmeal, smoothie bowls, apples, and bananas, or just eating with a spoon.

Total time: 15 minutes
Yield: 1½ cups

- 2 cups (226g) dry-roasted hazelnuts (see Tip)
- 3 to 4 tablespoons coconut sugar
- 3 tablespoons (16g) cacao powder
- ¼ teaspoon kosher salt

PUT the roasted hazelnuts in a high-powered blender (I use a Vitamix) or bowl of a food processor fitted with the metal blade. Process at medium-high speed for 5 to 8 minutes, scraping down the sides of the container as necessary until smooth and fluid. Your processing time might be shorter if you're using a high-powered blender, and could take a little longer and require more scraping in the food processor.

ONCE the hazelnuts have broken down completely and formed a smooth, fluid nut butter, add 3 tablespoons of the coconut sugar, the cacao powder, and salt.

PROCESS again for another 30 seconds to break down the coconut sugar and make sure everything is well incorporated. Taste and add the extra sugar, if desired. You can also add more salt, to taste.

TRANSFER the nut butter to a 12-ounce glass jar with a tight-fitting lid. Store in the pantry for up to 1 week or in the fridge for about 1 month.

Tip

If you only have raw hazelnuts, spread them on a baking sheet and roast at 325°F until golden brown around the edges and aromatic, about 10 minutes. Stir the nuts a few times during roasting. Slide the nuts onto a plate to cool completely; make sure they're cool before using!

Prep time: 10 minutes
Cook time: 30 minutes
Total time: 40 minutes
Yield: about 1½ cups

....

Scant 2 cups full-fat coconut milk (one 13½-ounce can)

¼ cup (85g) pure maple syrup (see Tip)

⅓ cup (48g) coconut sugar

1 teaspoon pure vanilla extract

½ teaspoon sea salt

Tip

Substitute honey for the maple syrup if you want, but if you do the sauce will not be vegan friendly.

SALTED CARAMEL SAUCE
PALEO • GRAIN-FREE • VEGAN • NUT-FREE • NO-BAKE • GLUTEN-FREE • DAIRY-FREE

Traditionally, caramel sauce is made by scalding water and sugar in a pan until superhot, and then pouring cream into it, where it bubbles all over the place. Although that method is quicker than my Paleo and vegan version, this one is a lot less dramatic. It takes a slow and steady 30 to 40 minutes to boil down the luscious salted caramel sauce, but doesn't require the constant eye that traditional caramel does. Once it's ready, you'll be hard pressed not to spoon it into your mouth. I love drizzling it over pies and cupcakes.

....

IN a medium, heavy-bottomed saucepan, combine the coconut milk, maple syrup, and coconut sugar. Bring to a boil over medium heat and then reduce to a simmer. Cook for 30 to 40 minutes, stirring frequently, until the sauce reaches about 220°F on a candy thermometer, or until it's a dark amber color, is thick enough to coat the back of a spoon, and has a syrupy texture.

REMOVE from the heat and stir in the vanilla and salt.

LET the sauce cool a little and then pour it into a jar without a lid to cool completely. When cool, screw the lid on the jar and refrigerate for up to 2 weeks.

SERVE the sauce cold, or warm it up a little in the microwave or on the stove over low heat.

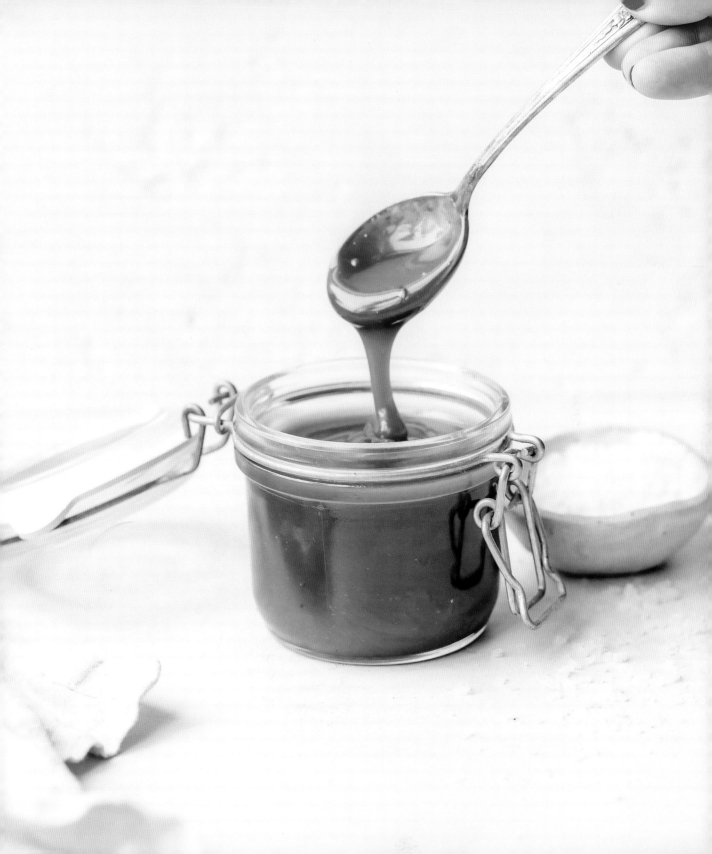

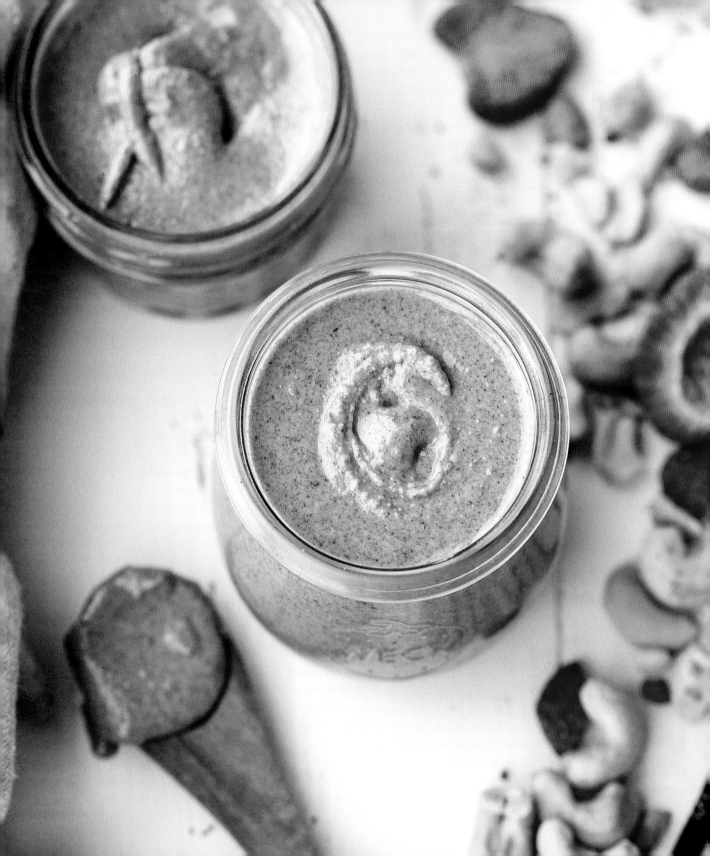

STRAWBERRY CASHEW BUTTER

PALEO • GRAIN-FREE • VEGAN • GLUTEN-FREE • DAIRY-FREE

This is a recipe I've had on my site for a few years, and I'm always trying to push it on people because once someone tries it . . . they're hooked. It's a game changer. Made with just cashews, freeze-dried strawberries, vanilla bean powder, and a bit of sea salt, it's so simple, but the flavors are magnificent. Buttery cashews with bright strawberry flavor and smooth vanilla bean . . . mmm. A jar of the butter makes a delicious and unique gift!

Prep time: 20 minutes
Bake time: 10 minutes
Total time: 30 minutes
Yield: 2 cups

2 cups (226g) raw cashews

¾ cup freeze-dried strawberries

1 teaspoon vanilla bean powder

¼ teaspoon sea salt

1 to 2 tablespoons refined coconut oil (if needed)

PREHEAT the oven to 350°F and line a baking sheet with parchment paper.

SPREAD the cashews on the baking sheet and bake for about 10 minutes, until fragrant and lightly toasted. Let the nuts cool for a few minutes on the baking sheet. (If you are short on time, you can leave the nuts raw, but they're easier to blend and more delicious when they've been toasted.)

WHEN the nuts are cool, transfer to the bowl of a food processor fitted with the metal blade or high-powered blender (I use a Vitamix). Process for 3 to 6 minutes, scraping down the sides of the bowl or blender as necessary, until the nuts are smooth and creamy. The nuts will process faster and require less scraping in the blender than in the food processor.

WHEN the cashews form a creamy butter, add the strawberries, vanilla, and salt. Process to incorporate. Taste the butter and adjust the ingredients according to your taste. Add coconut oil if the butter is too thick. (I usually add 1 tablespoon to make it a little bit drippy.)

TRANSFER the butter to one or two glass jars (such as mason or Weck jars). Cover the jars with their lids and store the butter at room temperature for up to 2 weeks, or in the refrigerator for up to 3 months.

Tip

For a quicker version of this recipe, replace the cashews with a 16-ounce jar of cashew butter and simply process the butter with the rest of the ingredients.

Prep time: 10 minutes
Bake time: 15 minutes
Total time: 25 minutes
Yield: about 2 cups

....

2½ cups (300g) raw cashews

2 to 3 tablespoons refined
    coconut oil

1 to 2 tablespoons coconut sugar

1 teaspoon vanilla extract, or
    ½ teaspoon vanilla bean
    powder

½ teaspoon ground cinnamon

¼ teaspoon kosher salt

¾ cup (81g) gluten-free rolled
    oats, toasted if you'd like
    (see Tips)

3 tablespoons cacao nibs or mini
    chocolate chips (see Tips)

OATMEAL-CHOCOLATE CHIP CASHEW BUTTER

PALEO • GRAIN-FREE • VEGAN • GLUTEN-FREE • DAIRY-FREE

Meet your new best friend! If you're a fan of oatmeal cookie dough by the spoonful, then this treat was made for you. Full of warm toasted oats and mini chocolate chips, it's far from your average nut butter. Make it extra thick and slather it on toast or between cookies, or thin it out and drizzle it on oatmeal, smoothie bowls, or ice cream. You can also just devour it my favorite way: by the spoonful.

....

PREHEAT the oven to 350°F. Line a baking sheet with parchment paper.

SPREAD the cashews on the baking sheet and roast for about 10 minutes, until fragrant and lightly toasted. Let the nuts cool for a few minutes on the baking sheet. (If you are short on time, you can leave the nuts raw, but they're easier to blend and taste better when they've been toasted.)

PUT the still-warm nuts in the bowl of a food processor fitted with the metal blade or in a high-powered blender (I use a Vitamix). Process for 3 to 6 minutes, scraping down the sides of the bowl and blender as necessary, until the nuts are smooth and creamy. The nuts will process faster and require less scraping in the blender than in the food processor.

WHEN the cashews have broken down into a smooth, creamy butter, add 2 tablespoons of the coconut oil, 1 tablespoon of the coconut sugar, the vanilla, cinnamon, and salt. Process to incorporate the ingredients. Taste the butter and adjust the ingredients as desired, adding more coconut sugar if you'd like it sweeter or more coconut oil if you'd like it thinner, or both. Add the oats and pulse to mix them in.

IF using the cacao nibs, add them now and pulse to mix. If you're using the mini chocolate chips, let the nut butter cool completely before adding them and pulsing to mix.

CONTINUES

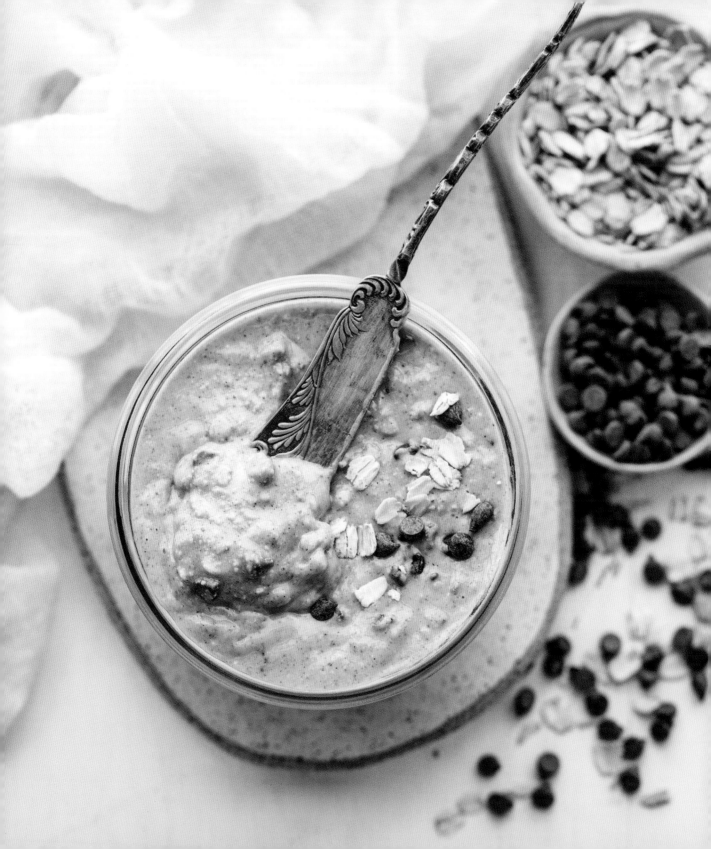

TRANSFER the butter to one or two glass jars (such as mason or Weck jars). Cover the jars with their lids and store the butter at room temperature for up to 2 weeks, or in the refrigerator for up to 3 months.

Tips

- To toast the oats, heat a medium nonstick skillet over medium heat. Add the oats and toast for 5 to 10 minutes, tossing them often, until they are lightly fragrant and light golden brown. Remove the oats from the skillet and let them cool on a plate.
- Substitute raisins for the chocolate chips to make oatmeal-raisin cashew butter!

NO-COOK CARAMEL SAUCE

PALEO • GRAIN-FREE • VEGAN • NO-BAKE • GLUTEN-FREE • DAIRY-FREE

So quick and easy to make, I love keeping a jar of this sauce in the fridge so I can drizzle caramel on anything at a moment's notice. It's made with a base of nut butter: My favorite is cashew butter because I find it has the most caramel-like taste, but any other nut butter can be used. Almond butter also tastes great, or use peanut butter for a peanut butter caramel!

Total time: 5 minutes
Yield: 1 generous cup

½ cup (128g) creamy cashew butter

⅓ cup (113g) pure maple syrup

⅓ cup (67g) refined coconut oil

¼ teaspoon sea salt

½ teaspoon vanilla extract

STIR together the cashew butter, maple syrup, and coconut oil. Microwave for 30 seconds, or until the ingredients melt together. Whisk to combine. Add the salt and vanilla and stir again. When well mixed, serve right away or pour the sauce into a jar with a tight-fitting lid.

KEEP the sauce, tightly covered, in the refrigerator for up to 1 month. It will firm up as it chills, so warm it in the microwave for about 30 seconds before using or spoon the sauce into a small saucepan and warm it over low heat until liquid.

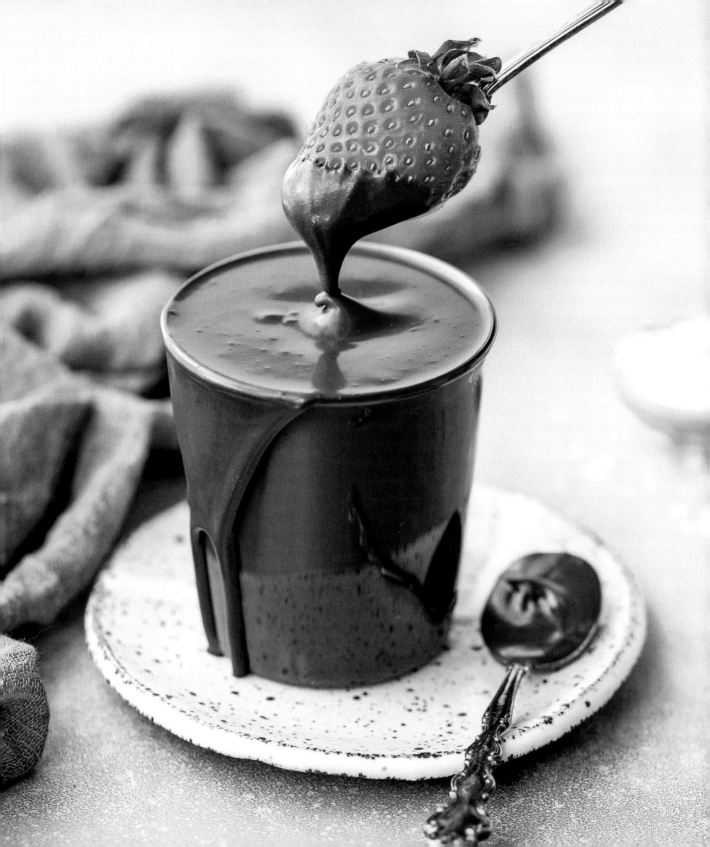

HOT FUDGE SAUCE

PALEO • GRAIN-FREE • VEGAN • NUT-FREE • NO-BAKE •
GLUTEN-FREE • DAIRY-FREE

Need the perfect thing to drizzle over your Double Chocolate Chunk Skillet Cookie (page 166) or Ultimate Fudge Brownies (page 201)? Look no further than this hot fudge—it's begging to be drizzled on anything where extra chocolate flavor is wanted. The smooth sauce is also perfect to use as a dip for fruit, pretzels, and whatever else you can think of.

Prep time: 5 minutes
Cook time: 10 minutes
Total time: 15 minutes
Yield: 1½ cups

1 cup canned full-fat coconut milk

¼ cup (21g) cocoa powder

¼ cup (36g) coconut sugar

2 tablespoons (25g) refined coconut oil

4 ounces bittersweet chocolate chips or chunks (about ⅔ cup)

1 teaspoon pure vanilla extract

Kosher salt

IN a medium saucepan, combine the coconut milk, cocoa powder, coconut sugar, and coconut oil. Bring to a boil, reduce the heat, and simmer for about 3 minutes, whisking frequently to melt the sugar and thicken the sauce slightly.

ADD the chocolate, vanilla, and salt to taste. Let the sauce sit for a minute to let the chocolate melt and then whisk until smooth and glossy. Let the sauce cool for 10 to 15 minutes before serving warm.

THE sauce will thicken when chilled. Heat in the microwave for 15 to 30 seconds or on the stove top, and stir the warm sauce before serving. To store, transfer the sauce to a jar with a tight-fitting lid and refrigerate for up to 1 week.

Total time: 10 minutes

Yield: 2 cups

2½ cups (283g) unsalted roasted peanuts

⅓ cup (58g) cacao butter, melted

2 tablespoons (18g) coconut sugar

1 cup gluten-free pretzels

WHITE CHOCOLATE–PRETZEL PEANUT BUTTER

VEGAN • NO-BAKE • GLUTEN-FREE • DAIRY-FREE

Before I was ever interested in vegetarian or vegan eating, there was a vegetarian restaurant I loved to frequent with my dad. Besides having a fun swing chair, I loved this spot because they had tons of flavors of house-made nut butter for sale in addition to a fantastic menu. The one I could never resist grabbing a jar of when we left was their white-chocolate-pretzel peanut butter: incredibly creamy, with the sweetness of white chocolate cut with the crunchy, salty flavor of pretzels. I've re-created those flavors with melted cacao butter, coconut sugar, and gluten-free pretzels, and it's just as good as I remember. This is a nut butter best served with a spoon, or as a dip for things like strawberries and apples!

PUT the peanuts in the bowl of a food processor fitted with the metal blade or a high-powered blender (I use a Vitamix) and process for 5 to 7 minutes, until the mixture is completely smooth. Scrape down the bowl and blender several times as necessary. Use the tamper for the blender to push the peanuts toward the blades. As the nuts are processed, they will go through stages: powdery, and then pasty, before the mixture turns into a big ball. Don't worry. As the oils are released, the nuts will continue to break down until the butter is creamy and delicious!

ONCE the mixture reaches a creamy consistency, add the melted cacao butter and coconut sugar and process until well mixed. Add the pretzels and pulse until the butter is smooth with a discernable crunch from the pretzels.

TRANSFER the butter to jars with tight-fitting lids. Refrigerate for up to 2 months, or keep at room temperature for up to 2 weeks.

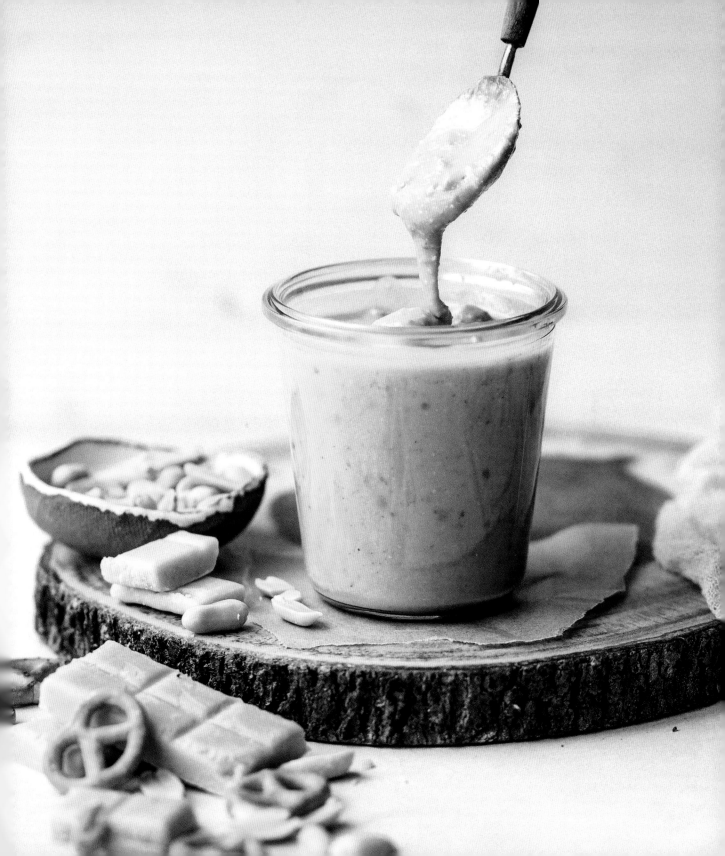

Index

Note: Page references in *italics* indicate photographs.

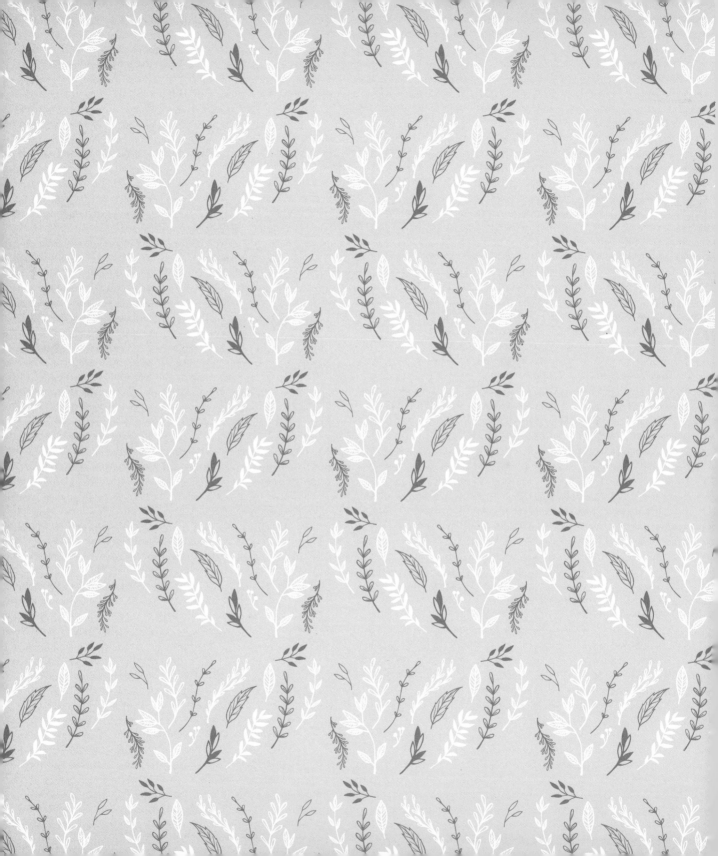